Arthur G. Lipman
Kenneth C. Jackson II
Linda S. Tyler
Editors

Evidence Based Symptom Control in Palliative Care: Systematic Reviews and Validated Clinical Practice Guidelines for 15 Common Problems in Patients with Life Limiting Disease

Evidence Based Symptom Control in Palliative Care: Systematic Reviews and Validated Clinical Practice Guidelines for 15 Common Problems in Patients with Life Limiting Disease has been co-published simultaneously as *Journal of Pharmaceutical Care in Pain & Symptom Control*, Volume 7, Number 4 1999 and Volume 8, Number 1 2000.

Pre-publication
REVIEWS,
COMMENTARIES,
EVALUATIONS . . .

"This innovative publication provides a long-awaited synopsis of highly organized and cogent symptom management information for clinicians at all stages of their careers caring for very ill patients. The voluble and repeated calls for empirical practice have, thankfully, germinated and born fruit through these authors' effort.

In view of the rapidly increasing numbers of people affected by far-advanced diseases this contribution should be celebrated as a giant step forward in this area of healthcare. If used as directed, there is every reason to believe that the results will be quite positive for patient and caregivers alike."

Perry G. Fine, MD
Professor, Pain Management Center
University of Utah
and
National Medical Director
VistaCare Hospice

More pre-publication
REVIEWS, COMMENTARIES, EVALUATIONS . . .

"**I**n the absence of excellent symptom management, it is impossible to provide effective hospice/palliative care. Dying persons typically experience multiple, progressive physical symptoms that confound caregivers, diminish the patient's quality of life, and frustrate everyone involved, especially the patient and family.

Most physicians are inadequately trained and inexperienced in the pharmacologic management of the physical symptoms commonly manifest in dying persons.

This thoroughly documented, rationally outlined and clearly written volume sets a new high standard of excellence for symptom management in palliative care. It offers science instead of conjecture and algorithms in place of guesswork. Moreover, it provides cost comparisons for various options, asks stimulating questions at the end of each section regarding further research and indicates the relative evidence supporting of each treatment option.

Evidence based treatment has come to palliative care. There is great reason to be grateful for the arrival of this book."

William M. Lamers Jr., MD
Medical Consultant
Hospice Foundation of America

"**T**here is a universal agreement of the urgent need for evidence based symptom management. This text addresses this priority concern for researchers and clinician in palliative care. The text is a valuable resource providing clear, concise information regarding common physical and pyschological symptoms at the end of life. For the clinician reader, the text provides an expert summary of key symptoms, pharmacologic treatment options and issues to guide treatment decision making. The text is also a superb resource for students and senior researchers in providing a review of current knowledge and clear direction for future research. The book's highlights include excellent tables summarizing the evidence of symptom management, reference lists for each symptom, cost data, and clinical prescribing information."

Betty Rolling Ferrell, PhD, FAAN
Research Scientist
City of Hope National Medical Center

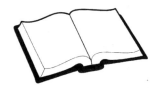

"This unique volume heralds the emergence of palliative care from the periphery of mainstream healhcare to its center. In preindustrial societies life is short, mortality high, and infection is the commonest cause of death. In industrialized nations mortality–particularly childhood mortality–declines, lifespan increases, and deaths from chronic illnesses such as heart disease and cancer soar. The increasingly knowledgeable, empowered and ageing populations of developed nations want healthcare that optimizes quality of life, recognizes patients' dignity and respects their values, and avoids futile and costly prolongation of life. Modern palliative care accepts scientific medicine yet balances it with a holistic, patient-centered approach. Lipman, Jackson and Tyler advance the practice and scientific credibility of palliative care by summarizing the best available evidence on treatment of 15 common symptoms in this setting. As co-chair of US federal guideline panels on pain control, and an editor of the recently formed Coherence Collaborative Review Group on Pain, Palliative and Supportive Care, I applaud their goal to formulate an evidence based practice of palliative care. They have, within the limitations of the available literature, not simply assembled a valuable, clinically-oriented compendium of best available evidence for current practice. Of equal or greater importance, they help to change the culture of palliative care practice by presenting their findings in concise, algorithmic form, highlighting gaps in the literature, and promoting a rigorous methodological foundation to develop future clinical evidence."

Daniel B. Carr, MD, FABPM
Saltonstall Professor of Pain Research
Departments of Anesthesia
and Medicine
Tufts University School of Medicine
New England Medical Center
Boston, MA

Evidence Based Symptom Control in Palliative Care: Systematic Reviews and Validated Clinical Practice Guidelines for 15 Common Problems in Patients with Life Limiting Disease

Evidence Based Symptom Control in Palliative Care: Systematic Reviews and Validated Clinical Practice Guidelines for 15 Common Problems in Patients with Life Limiting Disease has been co-published simultaneously as *Journal of Pharmaceutical Care in Pain & Symptom Control*, Volume 7, Number 4 1999 and Volume 8, Number 1 2000.

The *Journal of Pharmaceutical Care in Pain & Symptom Control* Monographic "Separates"

Below is a list of "separates," which in serials librarianship means a special issue simultaneously published as a special journal issue or double-issue *and* as a "separate" hardbound monograph. (This is a format which we also call a "DocuSerial.")

"Separates" are published because specialized libraries or professionals may wish to purchase a specific thematic issue by itself in a format which can be separately cataloged and shelved, as opposed to purchasing the journal on an on-going basis. Faculty members may also more easily consider a "separate" for classroom adoption.

"Separates" are carefully classified separately with the major book jobbers so that the journal tie-in can be noted on new book order slips to avoid duplicate purchasing.

You may wish to visit Haworth's website at . . .

http://www.haworthpressinc.com

. . . to search our online catalog for complete tables of contents of these separates and related publications.

You may also call 1-800-HAWORTH (outside US/Canada: 607-722-5857), or Fax 1-800-895-0582 (outside US/Canada: 607-771-0012), or e-mail at:

getinfo@haworthpressinc.com

Evidence Based Symptom Control in Palliative Care: Systematic Reviews and Validated Clinical Practice Guidelines for 15 Common Problems in Patients with Life Limiting Disease, edited by Arthur G. Lipman, PharmD, FASHP, Kenneth C. Jackson II, PharmD, and Linda S. Tyler, PharmD, FASHP (Vol. 7, No. 4, 1999 & Vol. 8, No. 1, 2000). *Through case studies and clinical research, this reliable reference offers medical professionals innovative recommendations and suggestions for drug therapies that will improve the lives of patients who are in pain due to life-threatening diseases. Evidence Based Symptom Control in Palliative Care provides you with guidelines for treatment that will help meet the patient's last wishes, improve the quality-of-life for patients and their families, and lessen physical and emotional pain. Examining ways to alleviate the various ailments that patients endure, such as depression and dyspnea as a result of a life-ending disease, this vital guide gives you the data you need in order to offer patients relevant care and meet their needs.*

Drug Use in Assisted Suicide and Euthanasia, edited by Margaret P. Battin, PhD, and Arthur G. Lipman, PharmD (Vol. 3, No. 3/4 & Vol. 4, No. 1/2, 1996). *Chosen as one of Doody's "Best Health Sciences Books" for 1996! "Many chapters, some written by opponents of assisted suicide and euthanasia and others by advocates of these practices, offer excellent discussions of multiple aspects of assisted suicide and euthanasia, creating deep awareness of the complex issues involved. The perspective of pharmacists, which has often been overlooked, provides insightful information about pharmacists' attitudes about the use of drugs intended to end the lives of terminally ill patients. Includes concrete and specific information about the actual practice of drug use in assisted suicide and euthanasia." (Canadian Family Physician)*

Evidence Based Symptom Control in Palliative Care: Systematic Reviews and Validated Clinical Practice Guidelines for 15 Common Problems in Patients with Life Limiting Disease

Arthur G. Lipman, PharmD, FASHP
Kenneth C. Jackson II, PharmD
Linda S. Tyler, PharmD, FASHP
Editors

Evidence Based Symptom Control in Palliative Care: Systematic Reviews and Validated Clinical Practice Guidelines for 15 Common Problems in Patients with Life Limiting Disease has been co-published simultaneously as *Journal of Pharmaceutical Care in Pain & Symptom Control*, Volume 7, Number 4 1999 and Volume 8, Number 1 2000.

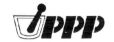

Pharmaceutical Products Press
An Imprint of
The Haworth Press, Inc.
New York • London • Oxford

Published by

Pharmaceutical Products Press®, 10 Alice Street, Binghamton, NY 13904-1580 USA

Pharmaceutical Products Press® is an imprint of The Haworth Press, Inc., 10 Alice Street, Binghamton, NY 13904-1580 USA.

Evidence Based Symptom Control in Palliative Care: Systematic Reviews and Validated Clinical Practice Guidelines for 15 Common Problems in Patients with Life Limiting Disease has been co-published simultaneously as *Journal of Pharmaceutical Care in Pain & Symptom Control*, Volume 7, Number 4 1999 and Volume 8, Number 1 2000.

Cover design by Thomas J. Mayshock Jr.

Library of Congress Cataloging-in-Publication Data

Evidence based symptom control in palliative care : systematic reviews and validated clinical practice guidelines for 15 common problems in patients with life limiting disease / Arthur G. Lipman, Kenneth C. Jackson II, Linda S. Tyler, editors.
      p. cm.–(Journal of pharmaceutical care in pain & symptom control; v. 7, no. 4-v. 8, no. 1)
      Includes bibliographical references and index.
      ISBN 0-7890-1013-5 (alk. paper)–ISBN 0-7890-1014-3 (alk. paper)
      1. Palliative treatment–Abstracts. 2. Terminal care–Psychology–Abstracts. 3. Evidence-based medicine–Abstracts. 4. Symptoms–Abstracts. I. Title: Systematic reviews and validated clinical practice guidelines for 15 common problems in patients with life limiting disease. II. Lipman, Arthur G. III. Jackson, Kenneth C. IV. Tyler, Linda S. V. Series.
      [DNLM: 1. Palliative Care–Abstracts. 2. Evidence-Based Medicine–Abstracts. 3. Terminal Care–psychology–Abstracts. ZWB 310 E93 2000]
R726.8.E93 2000
616'.029–dc21   00-032388

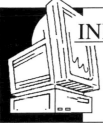

INDEXING & ABSTRACTING

Contributions to this publication are selectively indexed or abstracted in print, electronic, online, or CD-ROM version(s) of the reference tools and information services listed below. This list is current as of the copyright date of this publication. See the end of this section for additional notes.

- *Abstracts in Social Gerontology: Current Literature on Aging*

- *Adis International Ltd.*

- *AnalgesiaFile, Dannemiller Memorial Educational Foundation, Texas (www.pain.com)*

- *BUBL Information Service, an Internet-based Information Service for the UK higher education community. <URL:http://bubl.ac.uk/>*

- *CINAHL (Cumulative Index to Nursing & Allied Health Literature)*

- *CNPIEC Reference Guide: Chinese National Directory of Foreign Periodicals*

- *Current Contents . . . . . see: Institute for Scientific Information*

- *Derwent Drug File*

- *EMBASE/Excerpta Medica Secondary Publishing Division (URL:http://elsevier.nl)*

- *FINDEX (www.publist.com)*

- *Institute for Scientific Information*

- *International Pharmaceutical Abstracts*

- *Leeds Medical Information*

- *Pediatric Pain Letter*

- *Psychological Abstracts (PsycINFO)*

- *Referativnyi Zhurnal (Abstracts Journal of the All-Russian Institute of Scientific and Technical Information)*

(continued)

Special Bibliographic Notes related to special journal issues (separates) and indexing/abstracting:

- indexing/abstracting services in this list will also cover material in any "separate" that is co-published simultaneously with Haworth's special thematic journal issue or DocuSerial. Indexing/abstracting usually covers material at the article/chapter level.

- monographic co-editions are intended for either non-subscribers or libraries which intend to purchase a second copy for their circulating collections.

- monographic co-editions are reported to all jobbers/wholesalers/approval plans. The source journal is listed as the "series" to assist the prevention of duplicate purchasing in the same manner utilized for books-in-series.

- to facilitate user/access services all indexing/abstracting services are encouraged to utilize the co-indexing entry note indicated at the bottom of the first page of each article/chapter/contribution.

- this is intended to assist a library user of any reference tool (whether print, electronic, online, or CD-ROM) to locate the monographic version if the library has purchased this version but not a subscription to the source journal.

- individual articles/chapters in any Haworth publication are also available through the Haworth Document Delivery Service (HDDS).

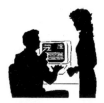

Evidence Based Symptom Control in Palliative Care: Systematic Reviews and Validated Clinical Practice Guidelines for 15 Common Problems in Patients with Life Limiting Disease

CONTENTS

Foreword: Format of the Clinical Practice Guidelines   xi
    Arthur G. Lipman

Preface   xiii
    Irene Higginson

Acknowledgments   xvii

Evidence-Based Palliative Care   1
    Arthur G. Lipman

Anorexia and Cachexia in Palliative Care Patients   11
    Linda S. Tyler
    Arthur G. Lipman

Anxiety in Palliative Care Patients   23
    Kenneth C. Jackson II
    Arthur G. Lipman

Bleeding Problems in Palliative Care Patients   37
    M. Christine Jamjian

Constipation in Palliative Care Patients   47
    M. Christina Beckwith

Delirium in Palliative Care Patients   59
   Kenneth C. Jackson II
   Arthur G. Lipman

Depression in Palliative Care Patients   71
   Andrew C. Martin
   Kenneth C. Jackson II

Diarrhea in Palliative Care Patients   91
   M. Christina Beckwith

Dyspnea in Palliative Care Patients   109
   Linda S. Tyler

Fatigue in Palliative Care Patients   129
   Linda S. Tyler
   Arthur G. Lipman

Oral Mucosal Problems in Palliative Care Patients   143
   Kenneth C. Jackson II
   Mark S. Chambers

Nausea and Vomiting in Palliative Care   163
   Linda S. Tyler

Nutrition and Hydration Problems in Palliative Care Patients   183
   Kenneth C. Jackson II

APPENDICES

Advances in Evidence-Based Information Resources
   for Clinical Practice   199
   R. Brian Haynes

The Cochrane Collaboration and Library: Accessing
   the Best Evidence Through Systematic Reviews   215
   Jeanne Le Ber

Index   229

ABOUT THE EDITORS

Arthur G. Lipman, PharmD, FASHP, is Professor in the College of Pharmacy, directs clinical pharmacology in the Pain Management Center and serves on the Pain Medicine and Palliative Care Advisory Group of the Huntsman Cancer Center at the University of Utah Health Sciences Center. He is a past president of the Utah State Cancer Pain Initiative, a member of the Board of Directors of the American Alliance of Cancer Pain Initiatives and a member of the Ethics Task Force of the American Pain Society American Academy of Pain Medicine. He was an investigator on the original National Cancer Institute-funded demonstration project of hospice care in Connecticut where he was on the faculty of the Yale University School of Medicine and Graduate School of Nursing. Dr. Lipman is a past president of Hospice of Salt Lake and was founding chair of the National Advisory Board of the Vista Hospice Care Foundation. He has several hundred publications and has made over 500 presentations at national and international professionals and scientific meetings. Dr. Lipman is the founding editor of the *Journal of Pharmaceutical Care in Pain & Symptom Control* and a past editor of the Research Update of the *American Pain Society Bulletin.*

Kenneth C. Jackson II, PharmD, is Manager for Clinical Pharmacy Services at St. Dominic–Jackson Memorial Hospital and on the clinical faculty at the University of Mississippi School of Pharmacy in Jackson, Mississippi. Dr. Jackson currently is Co-Chair of the Mississippi Cancer Pain Initiative. Prior to coming to Mississippi, Dr. Jackson completed a fellowship in pain management and palliative care research at the University of Utah in Salt Lake City, Utah and a specialty residency in nutritional support pharmacy practice at St. Mary Hospital in Lubbock, Texas.

Linda S. Tyler, PharmD, FASHP, is Professor at College of Pharmacy and Manager of Drug Information Services at University Hospitals and Clinics of the University of Utah Health Sciences Center. She currently serves on the United States Pharmacopeia Pharmacy Practice Advisory Panel and the American Society of Health-Systems Pharmacists Section of Clinical Specialists Board of Directors. She has published broadly and is a frequent invited speaker at national professional and scientific meetings on the topics of new drugs, statistics, research study design, drug information practice, formulary and outcomes management, and adverse drug reaction reporting.

Foreword:
Format of the Clinical Practice Guidelines

Evidence-Based Symptom Control in Palliative Care includes systematic reviews of the literature and validated clinical practice guidelines for 15 common problems in care of patients with advanced, irreversible disease. Systematically developed text, tables, and algorithms are presented in a consistent order for each symptom or symptom set. Evidence tables and drug therapy tables are provided. Additional tables are included for some symptoms when addition evidence was identified that was conducive to presentation as such.

These guidelines are designed to provide clinicians with clinical recommendations based on published evidence which have been validated through reviews and field testing by experienced palliative care clinicians. Because the literature describes some symptoms in pairs, six of the symptoms in this publication are discussed in sets, i.e., nausea and vomiting, anorexia and cachexia, nutrition and hydration problems.

Each symptom control guideline is formatted to include the following elements.

- Summary
- Keywords
- Algorithm (flow chart) more than one algorithm was necessary for some symptoms
- Literature review

[Haworth co-indexing entry note]: "Foroward: Format of the Clinical Practice Guidelines." Lipman, Arthur G. Co-published simultaneously in *Journal of Pharmaceutical Care in Pain & Symptom Control* (Pharmaceutical Products Press, an imprint of The Haworth Press, Inc.) Vol. 7, No. 4, 1999, and Vol. 8, No. 1, 2000, pp. xv-xvi; and: *Evidence Based Symptom Control in Palliative Care: Systematic Reviews and Validated Clinical Practice Guidelines for 15 Common Problems in Patients with Life Limiting Disease* (ed: Arthur G. Lipman, Kenneth C. Jackson II, and Linda S. Tyler) Pharmaceutical Products Press, an imprint of The Haworth Press, Inc., 2000, pp. xi-xii. Single or multiple copies of this article are available for a fee from The Haworth Document Delivery Service [1-800-342-9678, 9:00 a.m. - 5:00 p.m. (EST). E-mail address: getinfo@haworthpressinc. com].

xi

- Evidence tables
- Drug therapy tables
- Discussion of available evaluation instruments for the symptom(s) when available
- List of some open research questions
- References

By definition, this publication is a work in progress. New studies and observations will inevitably lead to changes in the recommendations. Periodic supplements to and revisions of these guidelines and additional guidelines will be published in the *Journal of Pharmaceutical Care in Pain & Symptom Control*. Information about the Journal is available from The Haworth Press, Inc., on the World Wide Web at www.haworthpressinc.com; by e-mail at getinfo@haworthpressinc.com; or by telephone at 800-895-0583.

Persons who review and use these guidelines are encouraged to communicate their experience with them, additional references, and suggested revisions (e-mail: alipman@pharm.utah.edu). No publication such as this is static. Continual refinement and revision is necessary if we are to provide optimal care to our patients.

Arthur G. Lipman

Preface

The use of evidence on which to base clinical practice has always been at the heart of palliative care. Early research in many countries had identified problems for patients and families towards the end of life. At that time, palliative care research was often unpopular and unrecognized in academic departments. In founding St. Christopher's Hospice, Dame Cicely Saunders wished to test which drugs were most appropriate in the control of pain and symptoms. She recognized that it is only by rigorously testing and analyzing which therapies work for which patients that we are able to improve the treatments we have an offer.

Therefore, it is particularly pleasing to introduce this publication gathering together an evidence-based approach to symptom control. This is a welcome addition to the many textbooks in all fields of medicine which delineate treatments but do not provide information on the evidence upon which these treatments are based. Here the authors have attempted to prepare the guidelines using research information. Although full detail of their literature reviews are not available, this publication represents an important step forward. Individuals reading it are informed of the basis upon which treatment decisions and recommendations, and can if they wish, agree or disagree with the assumptions made by the authors.

Systematic literature reviews aim to provide an unbiased approach to assembling the evidence by their systematic approach to locating, appraising and synthesizing research studies.[1] Studies are graded in a hierarchy according to the rigor of the study design. Of course, an

---

[Haworth co-indexing entry note]: "Preface." Higginson, Irene. Co-published simultaneously in *Journal of Pharmaceutical Care in Pain & Symptom Control* (Pharmaceutical Products Press, an imprint of The Haworth Press, Inc.) Vol. 7, No. 4, 1999, pp. xvii-xix; and: *Evidence Based Symptom Control in Palliative Care: Systematic Reviews and Validated Clinical Practice Guidelines for 15 Common Problems in Patients with Life Limiting Disease* (ed: Arthur G. Lipman, Kenneth C. Jackson II, and Linda S. Tyler) Pharmaceutical Products Press, an imprint of The Haworth Press, Inc., 2000, pp. xiii-xv. Single or multiple copies of this article are available for a fee from The Haworth Document Delivery Service [1-800-342-9678, 9:00 a.m. - 5:00 p.m. (EST). E-mail address: getinfo@haworthpressinc.com].

xiii

absence of evidence does not mean that something is not effective, but it does mean that we do not know.

There are two important limitations on the use of evidence as the basis for palliative care. First, quality of life is difficult to measure in palliative care patients–thus many studies exclude quality of life. Second, studies are often difficult to conduct on patients at the end of life, resulting in many studies evaluating treatments excluding patients towards the very end of life. This makes it difficult to extrapolate results of the studies to palliative care. In this volume the authors have sought information from a wide range of studies, including the randomized controlled trial (the gold standard of evaluative research, but unfortunately often excluding many palliative patients) and other designs (which often do include patients towards the end of life). The grading of the evidence is shown in the tables so that the reader can be clear on what strength the recommendation for treatment is made.

The practice of evidence-based care means integrating clinical expertise and findings with the best available external evidence from systematic research. Thus, the research findings and the guidelines presented here must be integrated with clinical experience and patient and family wishes. This includes considering total care, physical, emotional, social and spiritual, and including the family and lay carers as part of the unit of care. Greenhalgh[2] has identified eight questions to determine whether practice is evidence-based. These are adapted to incorporate palliative care and are:

1. Have I identified and prioritized the clinical, psychological, social and other problems, taking into account the patient and families perspective?
2. Have I performed a sufficiently competent and complete assessment (including examination) to establish the likelihood of competing diagnoses?
3. Have I considered additional problems and risk factors that may need opportunistic attention?
4. Have I, where necessary, sought evidence for systematic reviews, guidelines, clinical trials and other sources pertaining to the problem?
5. Have I assessed and taken into account the completeness, quality and strength of the evidence?

6. Have I applied valid and relevant evidence to the particular set of problems in a way that is both scientifically justified and intuitively sensible?
7. Have I presented the pros and cons of different options to the patient and family in a way that they can understand and incorporated the patient and family's wishes into the final recommendation?
8. Have I arranged review, recall, referral or further care as necessary?

This publication will be useful for all individuals who wish to develop evidence-based practice.

Irene Higginson, BMed Sci, BMBS, FFPHM, PhD
Professor and Head
Department of Palliative Care and Policy
King's College School of Medicine and Dentistry
University of London and
St. Christopher's Hospice
London, England

REFERENCES

1. Hearn J., Feuer D., Higginson D, Sheldon T. Systematic reviews. *Pall Med* 1999; 13:75-80
2. Greenhalgh T. Is my practice evidence based? *BMJ* 1996;313:957-958.

Acknowledgments

This publication is the culmination of over two years of searching and analyzing the literature, developing treatment recommendations, reviewing, field testing, and refining of the clinical practice guidelines which follow.

This work was supported in part by an unrestricted grant from the VistaCare Foundation. The editors express deep appreciation to the VistaCare Foundation and VistaCare Hospice programs throughout the United States for helping to make this publication possible.

The editors also express appreciation to the following individuals for their comments and suggestions during the development of these guidelines.

Ann Berger, MD
Diane Bowen, RN
Ira Byock, MD
Nessa Coyle, RN, MS
Charles Cleeland, PhD
Betty R. Ferrell, PhD, FAAN
Perry Fine, MD
Eric H. Frankle, PharmD
Barbara Franz, RN
Terrence Fleming, DDS
Myra Glajchen, DWS
William Lamers, MD
Jeanie Morris, RN
Steven Passik, PhD
Sharon Weinstein, MD

Evidence-Based Palliative Care

Arthur G. Lipman

SUMMARY. Palliative care and evidence-based medicine are defined and a brief history of modern hospice care is provided. Much palliative care provided today is based on anecdote, not evidence. While there are limited systematic reviews done in palliative care patients, there are sufficient small randomized controlled trials, n of 1 studies, and case reports to define clinical practice guidelines for common symptoms. The necessity for initiating palliative care as soon as possible after diagnosis of a life limiting disease is discussed. Symptom prevalence in palliative care patients is described. The process by which these guidelines were developed and the 5 levels of evidence are presented in a manner similar to that defined for the Agency for Health Care Policy and Research (AHCPR) clinical practice guideline on the management of cancer pain. Uses and limitations of the guidelines are described. *[Article copies available for a fee from The Haworth Document Delivery Service: 1-800-342-9678. E-mail address: getinfo@haworthpressinc.com <Website: http://www.haworthpressinc.com>]*

KEYWORDS. Palliative care, evidence-based medicine, dying, terminal care, symptoms, prevalence, initiation of care, physical, psychosocial, spiritual, existential, hospice, opium, opioids, systematic review

---

Arthur G. Lipman, PharmD, is Professor, College of Pharmacy, Director of Clinical Pharmacology, Pain Management Center, University Hospitals and Clinics; Pain Medicine and Palliative Care Advisory Group, Huntsman Cancer Center University of Utah Health Sciences Center, Salt Lake City, UT.

Address correspondence to: Arthur G. Lipman, PharmD, College of Pharmacy and Pain Management Center, 30 S 2000 E RM 258, University of Utah Health Sciences Center, Salt Lake City, UT 84112-5820 (E-mail: alipman@pharm.utah.edu).

[Haworth co-indexing entry note]: "Evidence-Based Palliative Care." Lipman, Arthur G. Co-published simultaneously in *Journal of Pharmaceutical Care in Pain & Symptom Control* (Pharmaceutical Products Press, an imprint of The Haworth Press, Inc.) Vol. 7, No. 4, 1999, pp. 1-9; and: *Evidence Based Symptom Control in Palliative Care: Systematic Reviews and Validated Clinical Practice Guidelines for 15 Common Problems in Patients with Life Limiting Disease* (ed: Arthur G. Lipman, Kenneth C. Jackson, II, and Linda S. Tyler) Pharmaceutical Products Press, an imprint of The Haworth Press, Inc., 2000, pp. 1-9. Single or multiple copies of this article are available for a fee from The Haworth Document Delivery Service [1-800-342-9678, 9:00 a.m. - 5:00 p.m. (EST). E-mail address: getinfo@haworthpressinc.com]

Algorithm for Key to Flow Chart Symbols

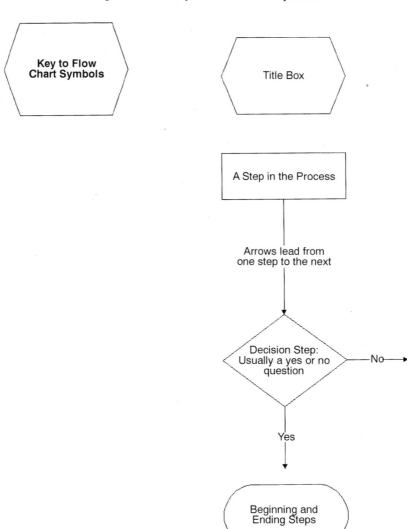

Palliative care has been defined and described by the World Health Organization as

> the active total care of patients whose disease is not responsive to curative treatment. Control of pain and other symptoms, and of psychological, social and spiritual problems is paramount. The goal of palliative care is achievement of the best quality of life for patients and their families. Many aspects of palliative care are also applicable earlier in the course of the illness in conjunction with (active treatment of the disease) . . . [1]

Evidence-based medicine has been defined as

> the conscientious, explicit and judicious use of current best evidence in making decisions about the care of individual patients.[2]

These two definitions appear logical and compatible. But evidence-based palliative care is more often the exception than the rule. Palliative care is largely based on anecdote and experience which often are not consistent with the evidence. This publication presents the evidence that has become available in recent years on the most effective and cost-effective management of 15 common symptoms experienced by patients with advanced, irreversible disease.

For thousands of years, opium, psychosocial interventions, and spiritual support have been mainstays of care of dying patients in pain. These frequently provided comfort, but did not extend life. The introduction in the latter half of the 20th century of medical techniques and drugs which often prolong life has shifted many clinicians' emphasis away from physical, psychological, social and spiritual support of patients with life threatening disorders. Tragically, this may lead to adverse outcomes. Recognition of that has led to the development of hospice and palliative care.

THE EVOLUTION OF MODERN PALLIATIVE CARE

Hospices were conceived in the middle ages as resting places for travelers. The first hospice identified specifically for care of the dying was established in 1842 in Lyon, France. In 1879, the Irish Sisters of Charity opened their first hospice in Dublin, and in 1899 Calvary Hospital was opened in New York City as a facility for care of terminally ill patients.

It was not until the latter decades of the 1900s that palliative care was redefined with the birth of the modern hospice movement.[3] Dame Cicely Saunders integrated her training as a nurse, a social worker, and a physician when, in 1967, she opened St. Christopher's Hospice in London. She defined dying patients' pain as physical, psychological and spiritual. The first hospice activity in North America began as a 1969 nursing study by Dean Florence Wald in New Haven[4] which led to the formation of the Connecticut Hospice in 1974.[5] Dr. Balfour Mount established the Palliative Care Unit at the Royal Victoria Hospital in Montreal a year later.

Newton's third law of motion teaches us about equal and opposite reactions. A pendulum at one extreme must go to the other extreme before it can settle in the middle. If one extreme is solely supportive care without ability to save life, the opposite extreme is aggressive–often futile–attempts to save life without attention to the dying patient's physical, emotional, and existential needs. Palliative care attempts to bring the pendulum into the center by defining scientifically valid, patient-specific care which addresses physical, psychosocial and existential needs of patients with limited life expectancies. To do so, palliative care must be introduced as soon as possible after the diagnosis of life limiting disease, *not* after life sustaining measures have been tried and judged futile. The current and optimal schema for the initiation of palliative care are illustrated in the following figure.

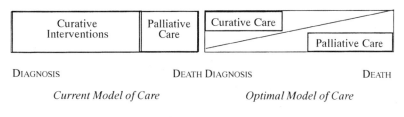

DIAGNOSIS   DEATH DIAGNOSIS   DEATH

Current Model of Care   *Optimal Model of Care*

Adapted from Reference 1

Good palliative care is being provided with increasing frequency. In the United States, the National Hospice Organization estimates that over 3,000 hospice programs now exist. But far too often, the palliative care provided is too little and too late.

BARRIERS TO PALLIATIVE CARE

Barriers to effective and timely provision of palliative care include physicians', nurses', pharmacists', and other health professionals' lack of knowledge; attitudes that every measure must be taken to extend life, even if such measures seriously erode the quality of remaining life; and the perception of death as failure of health care rather than the normal and inevitable process that it is. Many social and medical scientists, educators and policy makers are addressing these issues today.

One of the greatest barriers to optimal palliative care is the lack of evidence upon which to base it. Admittedly, it is far more difficult to study the effects of therapeutic interventions in palliative care patients than in the general population. The gold standard for studies of clinical interventions is the randomized controlled trial. Obvious ethical constraints preclude many randomized controlled trials being conducted with patients approaching the end of life. But some such data do exist. And it sometimes possible to extrapolate the results of studies conducted with healthier patients to palliative care patients. Good clinicians are good observers. Astute clinical observations and n of 1 studies also have added to the palliative care literature. The end result is that there is now some evidence upon which palliative care can and should be based.

This publication is a compilation of that literature and an attempt to place it into a clinically useful perspective. By definition, this is a work in progress. While 15 of the most common and troublesome symptoms experienced by palliative care patients are addressed, other such as cough, dysphagia, dysuria, and hiccups are not. Reports that we did not identify and that would augment this publication doubtless exist. This may be due in large part to the lack of indexing of the clinical and research literature using symptom control and palliative terms. Fortunately, that deficiency is now being corrected by members of the Pain and Palliative and Supportive Care (PaPaS) Collaborative Review Group of the International Cochrane Collaboration.[6]

EVIDENCE AND PALLIATIVE CARE

Numerous expert committee reports on symptom control have been developed by various national and international societies and agencies in recent years. Those reports are valuable because they reflect the opinions of knowledgeable experts. But they do not necessarily reflect the evidence. Only by seriously examining the evidence and then–when indicated–putting aside our personal biases and practices, will we be able to provide the most effective care for our patients.

Economic constraints are an unavoidable part of all health care. Capitated reimbursement, less than adequate governmental funding, and the rapidly escalating costs of new therapies place serious funding constraints on palliative care. It is essential that we provide not only effective, but cost-effective palliative care. Toward that end, this publication lists costs of drug therapy and suggests the least expensive of comparable therapies in the recommended treatments.

Individual studies provide potentially useful information. But only by reviewing the body of literature on a subject as a whole can we gain a true perspective on what is known–and not known. Systematic reviews have been defined as integrative articles based on evidence synthesized from a comprehensive literature search from which selected articles are taken according to predefined criteria.[7] Systematic reviews present the extant data in such a format. The reviews that follow also helped the authors to identify open research questions, some of which are listed for each symptom.

The model for this work was the evidence based clinical practice guideline entitled Management of Cancer Pain which was published in 1994 by the Agency for Health Care Policy and Research (AHCPR) of the Public Health Service, U.S. Department of Health and Human Services.[8] (A revision of that guideline was in preparation at the time of this writing by the Clinical Practice Guidelines Committee of the American Pain Society.[9])

The 1994 guideline was developed as "a synthesis of the scientific research and expert judgement to make recommendations on pain assessment and management." Extensive literature searches were followed by meta-analyses of those randomized controlled trials that met stringent acceptance criteria, best evidence synthesis from all levels of evidence, and these extensive reviews, revisions and field testing of the guideline to assure both internally and externally validity. The five evidence levels that defined in the AHCPR process were adapted for use in the development of these evidence based guidelines as follows.

Level I	Randomized trials with low false-positive (alpha) and low false-negative (beta errors); high power;
Level II	Randomized trials with high false-positive (alpha) and/or high false-negative (beta errors); low power;
Level III	Nonrandomized concurrent cohort comparisons between contemporaneous patients who did and did not receive a given intervention;
Level IV	Nonrandomized historical cohort comparisons between current patients who did receive the intervention and patients (from the same institution or from the literature) who did not; and
Level V	Case series without control subjects.

SYMPTOM PREVALENCE

Several studies have defined the most common symptoms experienced by dying patients. The earlier studies involved primarily cancer patients. Palliative care today includes patients with many other diagnoses, e.g., dementia, congestive heart failure, end stage renal and hepatic disease, multiple sclerosis, amyotrophic lateral sclerosis, acquired immune deficiency syndrome, chronic pulmonary disease. Therefore, the range of symptoms experienced by these patients is increasing.

One of the more comprehensive reports of symptom prevalence in palliative care resulted from a multicenter study conducted in Spain during 1994.[10] It included 176 consecutive patients (mean age 67.7 years) who were evaluated at time of admission to hospital, home care or hospice and again within the last week of life. Two-thirds of the patients had metastatic disease; 52% of whom had multiple metastases. Presence, not severity, of symptoms was recorded and reported as follows.

Symptoms	Symptom Prevalence at Time of Admission to the Study	Symptom Prevalence One Week Before Death
	n (%)	*n (%)*
aesthenia	135 (76.7)	144 (81.8)
anorexia	120 (68.2)	141 (80.0)
dry mouth	108 (61.4)	123 (69.9)
confusion	53 (30.1)	120 (68.2)
constipation	87 (49.4)	97 (55.1)
dyspnea	70 (39.8)	82 (46.6)
dysphagia	49 (27.8)	81 (46.0)
anxiety	89 (50.6)	80 (45.5)
depression	93 (52.8)	68 (38.6)
paralysis	36 (20.5)	57 (32.4)
pain	92 (52.3)	53 (30.1)
sleep disturbance	61 (34.7)	50 (28.8)
cough	49 (27.8)	31 (17.6)
nausea	46 (26.1)	23 (13.1)
hemorrhage	28 (15.9)	21 (11.8)
vomiting	33 (18.8)	18 (10.2)
diarrhea	16 (9.1)	12 (6.8)
dysuria	14 (8.0)	12 (6.8)

APPLYING THE EVIDENCE TO PATIENT CARE

The practice of evidence based medicine means integrating individual clinical expertise with the best available clinical evidence in making decisions about individual patients. It should lead to thoughtful identification and compassionate use of individual patients' problems and preferences in making clinical decisions. Evidence-based medicine is not "cookbook" medicine. Evidence can inform, it cannot replace individual clinical expertise and patients' choices.[2]

Readers are discouraged from using the clinical recommendations listed in the text and algorithms of this publication without carefully considering how the recommendations apply to the specific patient for whom care is being planned.

USING THE ALGORITHMS

The algorithms included with these guidelines are attempts at integrating the evidence in palliative care patients with existing knowledge about the drug therapy and extensive clinical experience of the authors and reviewers. The algorithms do not necessarily define the most appropriate treatment for any given patient. They represent approaches to care that should be adjusted according to individual patient needs. By definition, these algorithms are products of best evidence synthesis. For more than half of the symptoms addressed, the existing evidence is modest.

The meaning of the symbols in the algorithms is as follows.

It is the intent and hope of all involved in the development, review and validation of this publication that the evidence and recommendations provided will allow clinicians to improve their patients' clinical outcomes and quality of remaining life.

REFERENCES

1. Cancer Pain Relief and Palliative Care. Report of a WHO Expert Committee. (Technical Report Series 804). Geneva, World Health Organization, 1990.

2. Sackett DL, Rosenberg WMC, Gray JAM, Haynes RB, Richardson WS. Evidence based medicine: what it is and what it isn't. BMJ 1996;312:71-2.

3. Twycross RG. Hospice care-redressing the balance in medicine. J Royal Soc Med. 1980;73:475-81.

4. Lipman AG. Drug therapy in terminally ill patients. Amer J Hosp Pharm 1975;32:270-6.

5. Friedrich MJ. Hospice care in the United States: a conversation with Florence S. Wald. JAMA 1999;281:1683-5.

6. http://www.jr2.ox.ac.uk/Cochrane/

7. Cook DJ, Greengold NL, Ellrodt AG Weingarten SR. The relationship between systematic reviews and practice guidelines. Ann Intern med 1997;127:210-6.

8. Jacox A, Carr DB, Payne R et al. Management of Cancer Pain. Clinical Practice Guideline. AHCPR Publication Number 94-0592, Rockville MD. Agency for Health Care Policy and Research, U.S. Department of Health and Human Services, Public Health Service, 1994.

9. http://www/ampainsoc.org

10. Conill C, Verger E, Henríquez I, et al. Symptom prevalence in the last week of life. J Pain Symptom Manage 1997;14:328-331.

Anorexia and Cachexia
in Palliative Care Patients

Linda S. Tyler
Arthur G. Lipman

SUMMARY. Anorexia and cachexia are common in patients with advanced degenerative diseases. Cachexia is especially problematic in AIDS patients. These symptoms often result from or are exacerbated by other symptoms such as nausea and constipation. Potential causes and supportive care are described. Drug therapy that has been used is summarized. Evaluation instruments that have been used for this symptom are described. Some open research questions are listed. Evidence tables and drug therapy tables which include drug costs are presented. *[Article copies available for a fee from The Haworth Document Delivery Service: 1-800-342-9678. E-mail address: getinfo@haworthpressinc.com <Website: http://www.haworthpressinc.com>]*

KEYWORDS. Anorexia, cachexia, appetite, weight loss, palliative care, terminal care, dying, supportive care, drug therapy, non-pharmacological therapy, etiology, evidence, corticosteroids, hydrazine, megestrol, pentoxifylline, cannabinoids, metoclopramide, cyproheptadine, costs, algorithm, systematic review

Linda S. Tyler, PharmD, is Professor, College of Pharmacy; and Manager, Drug Information Service, Department of Pharmacy Services, University Hospitals and Clinics; University of Utah Health Sciences Center, Salt Lake City, UT.

Arthur G. Lipman, PharmD, is Professor, College of Pharmacy; Director of Clinical Pharmacology, Pain Management Center, University Hospitals and Clinics; Pain Medicine and Palliative Care Advisory Group, Huntsman Cancer Center; University of Utah Health Sciences Center, Salt Lake City, UT.

Address correspondence to: Arthur G. Lipman, PharmD, College of Pharmacy and Pain Management Center, 30 S 2000 E RM 258, University of Utah Health Sciences Center, Salt Lake City, UT 84112-5820 (E-mail: alipman@pharm.utah.edu).

[Haworth co-indexing entry note]: "Anorexia and Cachexia in Palliative Care Patients." Tyler, Linda S., and Arthur G. Lipman. Co-published simultaneously in *Journal of Pharmaceutical Care in Pain & Symptom Control* (Pharmaceutical Products Press, an imprint of The Haworth Press, Inc.) Vol. 7, No. 4, 1999, pp. 11-22; and: *Evidence Based Symptom Control in Palliative Care: Systematic Reviews and Validated Clinical Practice Guidelines for 15 Common Problems in Patients with Life Limiting Disease* (ed: Arthur G. Lipman, Kenneth C. Jackson II, and Linda S. Tyler) Pharmaceutical Products Press, an imprint of The Haworth Press, Inc., 2000, pp. 11-22. Single or multiple copies of this article are available for a fee from The Haworth Document Delivery Service [1-800-342-9678, 9:00 a.m. - 5:00 p.m. (EST). E-mail address: getinfo@haworthpressinc.com].

Algorithm for Managing Anorexia and Cachexia

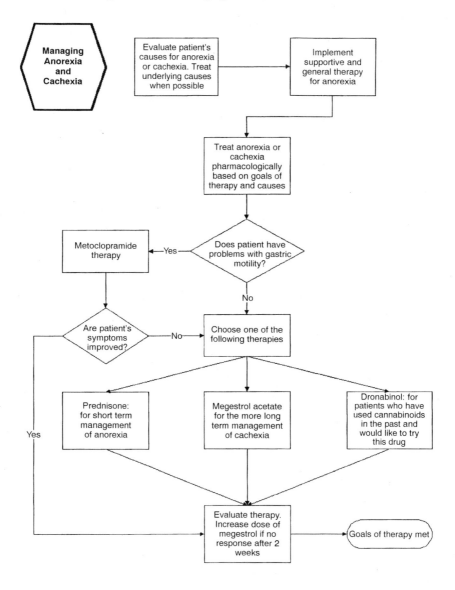

Several mechanisms associated with anorexia and cachexia in palliative care have been identified resulting in a range of recommendations for treatment.[1-6] Anorexia and cachexia are frequent in terminally ill patients. Table 1 summarizes the evidence on managing anorexia and cachexia with pharmacologic interventions. The following summarizes a treatment strategy for managing these patients and selecting appropriate pharmacologic agents.

Each patient with anorexia or cachexia should be evaluated and potential causes and contributing factors ascertained.

TREAT THE UNDERLYING CAUSE WHEN POSSIBLE

When possible, the underlying cause of the symptoms should be treated. Frequent causes of anorexia that can be treated include:

- Nausea and vomiting
- Constipation
- Dehydration
- Weakness
- Depression
- Pain
- Oral candidiasis or dry mouth
- Gastritis

IMPLEMENT SUPPORTIVE THERAPY

Many non-pharmacologic measures can be implemented to treat anorexia. These could include any of the following:

- Remove unpleasant odors.
- Treat pain optimally.
- Give an alcoholic drink prior to meals.
- Give small, frequent meals.
- Serve meals in a room besides where the patient sleeps.
- Provide companionship for patient with meals.
- Involve patient in menu planning.

TREAT ANOREXIA OR CACHEXIA PHARMACOLOGICALLY

Several pharmacologic agents have been recommended to improve patient's appetites and promote weight gain. These are summarized in Table 2.

TABLE 1. Drug Therapy for Managing Anorexia and Cachexia in Palliative Care Evidence Tables

Reference	Study Design	n	Intervention	Results	Level of Evidence	Comments
Corticosteroids						
Moertel (1974)[8]	Randomized double-blind	116	Patients with unresectable gastrointestinal adenocarcinoma received placebo, dexamethasone 0.75 mg qid, or dexamethasone 1.5 mg qid. Therapy continued until patient's death or unable to take oral medications.	Patients on dexamethasone reported improved appetite and improved strength. However, survival and weight gain was similar to placebo.	II	
Bruera (1985)[7]	Randomized double-blind	40	Patients who were terminally ill were randomized to receive methylprednisolone 16 mg po bid or placebo for 5 days, then crossed over to 5 days of the alternate therapy after a 3 day washout interval. After the crossover, all patients received 16 mg bid methylprednisolone.	31 patients completed the trial. Patients who received methylprednisolone demonstrated significant improvement in pain depression, appetite and food consumption. No change was noted on anxiety and performance status.	II	All nutritional parameters returned to baseline after the 20 days of therapy.
Popiela (1989)[9]	Randomized double-blind	173	Female cancer patients who were terminally ill received methylprednisolone 125 mg IV qd or placebo for 56 days.	Patients demonstrated significantly improved quality of life, including increased appetite, sense of well-being.	II	Groups demonstrated equal mortality and adverse effects.
Twycross (1985)[10]	Randomized double-blind	27	Patients with terminal cancer received prednisolone 5 mg po tid versus placebo for 7 days.	While patients on prednisolone demonstrated improved mood, sleep, and appetite, the difference was not significant.	II	
Schnell (1972)[11]	Follow-up study	315	Terminally ill patients with cancer who received steroids (n = 180) were compared with those who did not (n = 135) study examined differences via adverse effects.	Patients had five-times the risk of peptic ulcer. No other differences in adverse effects were noted.	IV	

Pentoxifylline (Trental)				
Goldberg (1995)[19]	Randomized double-blind	70	Patients with cancer related cachexia or anorexia were randomized to receive pentoxifylline 400 mg tid or placebo.	No benefit of pentoxifylline was identified, nor were any adverse effects.	=
Cannabinoids				
Nelson (1994)[18]	Descriptive	18	Patients treated in a palliative care unit with greater than a 4 week life expectance with anorexia received dronabinol 2.5 mg tid (bid if > 65 yr or older initially, increasing to tid after 3 days.) Patients received therapy for 28 days.	13 of 18 patients reported improved appetite; 10 reported slight improvement, 3 had major.	>
Cyproheptadine (Periactin)				
Kardinal (1990)[20]	Randomized double-blind	295	Patients with cancer were randomized to receive cyproheptadine 8 mg po tid (n = 143) or placebo (n = 150).	Patients on cyproheptadine had less nausea and emesis, but more sedation and dizziness. However, the weight loss was comparable to placebo.	=
Hydrazine Sulfate				
Chlebowski (1987)[22]	Randomized double-blind	101	Patients with advanced cancer received hydrazine sulfate 60 mg po tid, or placebo. Patients were treated for 30 days.	Weight was increased or maintained in 83% of the hydrazine patients compared to 53% of the placebo patients.	I
Chlebowski (1990)[21]	Randomized double-blind	65	Patients with non-small cell lung cancer receiving chemotherapy received hydrazine sulfate 60 mg po tid or placebo.	Caloric intake was significantly increased in hydrazine group. Weight loss was the same in both groups. Survival was greater in the hydrazine patients (292 days) compared to placebo (187 days), though not statistically significant.	=

TABLE 1 (continued)

Reference	Study Design	n	Intervention	Results	Level of Evidence	Comments
Megestrol Acetate (Megace)						
Loprinzi (1990)[15]	Randomized Double-blind	133	Cancer patients were randomized to receive placebo or megestrol acetate po 800 mg/d (320 mg on arising, 320 mg midday, and 160 mg at evening meal). Patients who lost 5% of their body weight during the trial had their treatment unblinded and were crossed over to megestrol therapy if they were on placebo.	16% of megestrol patients gained 15 lbs or more during the study compared to placebo 2% (p < 0.003). Megestrol patients reported more frequently improved appetite (p = 0.003) and food intake (p = 0.009) compared to placebo. 15 patients crossed over to megestrol therapy. The average weight loss in this patients was 6.2 lb/month on placebo compared to 0.5 lb/month on megestrol (p = 0.03).	I	Duration of therapy not specified in protocol. Patients received a median of 1.6 months of therapy. 49 patients received therapy for 10 weeks or longer. Patients were assessed monthly.
Loprinzi (1993)[14]	Randomized	342	Patients with cancer related anorexia or cachexia received megestrol acetate po. Patients were randomized to the following doses 160, 480, 800, or 1,280 mg. Patients had a life expectancy greater than 3 months. Patients were followed a median of 66 days.	While not statistically significant, a trend of increased dose and increased weight was noted (% of patients with >10% weight gain = 8%, 8%, 15%, 13%) Increased appetite was positively correlated with weight gain.	I	Higher dose (1,280 mg) offered no advantages compared to 800 mg dose.
Gebbia (1996)[13]	Randomized double-blind	122	Cancer patients with cachexia or anorexia were randomized to receive megestrol acetate 160 mg PO daily or 160 mg PO q12h. Patients were evaluated every 2 weeks. If after one month of therapy pt. did not demonstrate an increase in weight and appetite, the dose was increased to 320 mg/d or 480 mg/d, respectively.	An increase in weight was noted in 27% vs. 40% of patients at the lower doses, respectively after 15 days of therapy. After dosage increases, 18% of 320 mg patients had increase weight and 10% of the 480 mg group. Increased appetite was reported in 36% and 20% of patients, respectively.	I	Authors recommend start dose at 160 mg/d and increase if no response. Pt. response was noted at 2 weeks.

Oster (1994)[12]	Randomized double-blind	100	Patients with AIDS and cachexia were randomized to receive megestrol acetate 800 mg/d po or p acebo for 12 weeks.	Patients receiving megestrol acetate demonstrated significant weight gain (mean = 4.77 kg, CI95 = 2.06-7 48 kg) and increased sense of well being.	II
Loprinzi (1993)[14]	Descriptive	12	Patients receiving megestrol acetate 800 mg/d for treatment of anorexia or cachexia had body composition measurements at 2 month intervals after starting therapy.	Weight gain observed was due to an increase in body mass, mostly adipose. Increase in body fluid accounted for a small amount of the weight gain.	V
Ackerman (1993)[23]	Descriptive	15	Patients with advanced metastatic cancer receiving interferon α2b were given megestrol acetate po 60 mg/d (30 mg in a.m., 15 mg at noon, 15 mg at night.) Patients were evaluated at 4 weeks.	Only 10 pts. were evaluated. In the month prior to therapy, patients averaged 6.6% weight loss. After one month of therapy, patients had a mean 0.8% weight gain.	V
Pimentel ('996)[17]	Descriptive	1	Patient receive megestrol acetate 400 mg po daily for 5 days prior to presenting with hyperglycemia (1,039 mg/dL).	Symptoms resolved after discontinuing drug.	V
Walsh (1995)[24]	Descriptive	1	Patient with advanced cancer received megestrol acetate 80 mg bid.	Pt. demonstrated increased weight and appetite. Dose was decreased to 40 mg qd 3 months later because of excessive weight gain, and later to 40 mg bid.	V	Author advocates trying a lower dose and increasing dose based on this case and high drug cost.

Key to Level of evidence classification:

Level I   Randomized trials with low false-positive (alpha) and low false-negative (beta errors); high power
Level II   Randomized trials with high false-positive (alpha) and/or high false-negative (beta errors); low power
Level III Nonrandomized concurrent cohort comparisons between contemporaneous patients who did and did not receive a given intervention
Level IV Nonrandomized historical cohort comparisons between current patients who did receive intervention and patients (from the same institution or from the literature) who did not
Level V   Case series without control subjects

TABLE 2. Drug Therapy for Managing Cachexia and Anorexia in Palliative Care

Drug Therapy	Indications for Use	Dosing Regimen	AWP per Day of Therapy#
megestrol acetate (Megace)	Clinical trials demonstrate that patients have increased weight gain, appetite, and sense of well-being. Indicated for the more long-term management of cachexia.	160-800 mg po qd (available as 40 mg tablets) 160-800 mg po qd (available as 40 mg/mL suspension)	$3.42-17.00 $1.76-8.80
corticosteroids	Clinical trials report that patients demonstrate increased appetite and sense of well-being. Indicated when short-term therapy to increase appetite and sense of well-being is beneficial. May be especially useful in patients who have other reasons to take corticosteroids, such as bone pain or bronchospasm.	dexamethasone 2-4 mg po bid or tid (tablets) 2-4 mg po bid or tid (0.5 mg/5 mL elixir) prednisone 10-20 mg po qd or bid methylprednisolone 16 mg po bid	$1.16-1.75 $1.90-5.70 $0.03-0.13 $1.83
dronabinol (Marinol)	Clinical trials demonstrate a benefit of increased weight gain. Many patients do not tolerate the CNS effects. For patients who have liked marijuana in the past, this may be beneficial. Others may want to try it, but should be started at the lower dose.	2.5 mg po bid-tid	$5.78-8.67
metoclopramide (Reglan)	While no clinical trials support its use specifically in the management of anorexia and cachexia, many recommend it especially if there is an element of gastric stasis in the patient's symptoms. Some administer metoclopramide by continuous SQ infusion.[26,27]	10-20 mg po q6h 10-20 mg IV q6h	$0.08-0.15 $4.56-9.12
cyproheptadine (Periactin)	No clinical trials support its use, though some believe it may be worth trying in patients who have failed other therapies or cannot tolerate therapy.	4-8 mg po tid	$0.06 - 0.12

Average Wholesale Price, 1999 (cost to pharmacy)

18

Corticosteroids have also been studied in randomized, double-blind studies.[7-10] In general, corticosteroids improved patients' well-being and increased appetite, but did not cause weight gain. The effect of corticosteroids have not been evaluated in a long term (greater than 2 months) studies. These may be useful early on as an appetite stimulant when managing anorexia or if patient has a short life expectancy. Because of the low cost, some suggest using these as first line.

No differences in mortality between patients taking steroids and matched controls have been reported. In one series, patients receiving corticosteroids had more problems with gastrointestinal effects and cardiovascular effects than placebo patients.[9] Schnell[11] noted increased incidence of asymptomatic peptic ulcer disease on autopsy in patients who died from cancer receiving corticosteroids prior to death (10%) compared to placebo (2%). No other significant differences were identified between the groups.

Several randomized double-blind trials have evaluated megestrol acetate in patients with demonstrated weight loss.[12-16] Most of the studies have been conducted in cancer patients.[12-15] While the definitions vary among the studies, each selected a patient population with demonstrated weight loss in the previous month. Megestrol acetate results in weight gain, increased appetite, and increased sense of well-being while patients were taking the drug. The effect was sustained in patients who took the drug for a longer time interval.

Von Roenn et al.[16] reviewed two trials of using megestrol in AIDS-associated anorexia.

(*Editors' Note:* The original reports of these trials were not available for review and therefore are not included in the evidence tables. Doses used in the initial trial were 800 mg/d; the second trial used 100, 400, and 800 mg doses.)

The most effective initial dose is not clear. Loprinzi et al.[14] evaluated megestrol doses of 160, 480, 800, and 1,280 mg and found the greatest effect with 800 mg. No increased efficacy was noted at the higher dose. At the lower doses, a clear dose response relationship exists: the higher the dose, the greater the weight gain demonstrated. Others have demonstrated efficacy (weight gain) at lower doses (160-320 mg).[13] If patients are going to respond to therapy, a response is observed quickly, within 2 weeks. If patients do not respond to a given dose, the dose may be increased with many patients responding to the increased dose.

Adverse effects noted with megestrol acetate therapy included peripheral edema (10-19%),[13,15] venous thrombosis (6%),[13] nausea (3-12%),[15] menstrual irregularities (0-4%),[15] and impotence (19-33%).[15] Hyperglycemia has also been reported.[17] In Von Roenen et al.'s review,[16] rash (5.9%), dyspnea (2.9%), alopecia (1.1%), hyperglycemia (1.9%), deep vein thrombosis (0.3%), diarrhea (10%), and impotence (5.1%) were reported. Many of the adverse effects did not appear to be dose related in the studies that used several doses. No differences in survival were noted in these studies.

Many patients report a benefit from dronabinol therapy.[18] However, many are unable to tolerate the CNS adverse effects.

In one review article,[3] metoclopramide is recommended as first line therapy in patients with cancer related anorexia-cachexia syndrome. Based on its pharmacology, this drug would be most useful in patients with gastric stasis or other motility problems. No studies have evaluated its effectiveness in cachexia per se, or its role in palliative care.

Pentoxifylline was studied in one randomized double-blind trial, but no clinical benefit was identified.[19]

Cyproheptadine was thought to have a role in the management of anorexia and cachexia because of its anti-serotonergic effects. In one clinical trial,[20] patients experienced less nausea and emesis, but they also experienced more sedation and dizziness. Weight loss was the same as the placebo group.

Hydrazine sulfate has also been evaluated.[21,22] It is currently an investigational agent. Interest in hydrazine is based on its ability to inhibit gluconeogenesis, with resulting improvement in glucose and protein metabolism, and increased weight and albumin levels. Based on these initial trials, hydrazine may show promise in this setting. More trials are in progress to evaluate the more long term effects of using this agent.

EVALUATION OF ANOREXIA AND CACHEXIA

While many studies evaluate anorexia and cachexia in clinical trials, each often uses a different instrument to evaluation the patient's symptoms. A standardized approach to evaluating these symptoms would be helpful. The following reference is the only one that discusses an evaluation tool that was identified in the literature search.

Cella DF, VonRoenn J, Lloyd S, et al. The Bristol-Myers Anorexia/Cachexia Recovery Instrument (BACRI): A brief assessment of patients' subjective response to treatment for anorexia/cachexia. Qual Life Res 1995; 4:221-231.

SOME OPEN RESEARCH QUESTIONS

1. What is the most effective doses of megestrol acetate for management of anorexia and cachexia?
2. In what situations are corticosteroids indicated?
3. How much of a problem are adverse effects with these drugs?
4. Are there other studies that should be included in this analysis?
5. What patients might benefit from cyproheptadine?
6. What is the role of combination therapy?
7. How do corticosteroids compare with megestrol acetate therapy?

REFERENCES

1. Vigano A, Watanabe S, Bruera E. Anorexia and cachexia in advanced cancer patients. Cancer Surv. 1994;21:99-115.

2. Bruera E. Is the pharmacological treatment of cancer cachexia possible? Support Care Cancer. 1993;1:298-304.

3. Nelson KA, Walsh D, Sheehan FA. The cancer anorexia-cachexia syndrome. J Clin Oncol. 1994;12:213-25.

4. Plata-Salaman CR. Anorexia during acute and chronic disease. Nutrition. 1996;12:69-78.

5. Kotler DP, Grunfeld C. Pathophysiology and treatment of the AIDS wasting syndrome. AIDS Clin Rev. 1995;96:229-75

6. Splinter TA. Cachexia and cancer: a clinician's view. Ann Oncol. 1992;3: S25-S27.

7. Bruera E, Roca E, Cedaro L, Carraro S, Chacon R. Action of oral methylprednisolone in terminal cancer patients: a prospective randomized double-blind study. Cancer Treat Rep. 1985;69:751-4.

8. Moertel CG, Schutt AJ, Reitemeier RJ, Hahn RG. Corticosteroid therapy of preterminal gastrointestinal cancer. Cancer. 1974;33:1607-9.

9. Popiela T, Lucchi R, Giongo F. Methylprednisolone as palliative therapy for female terminal cancer patients. Eur J Cancer Clin Oncol. 1989;25:1823-9.

10. Twycross RG, Guppy D. Prednisolone in terminal breast and bronchogenic cancer. Practitioner. 1985;229:57-9.

11. Schell HW. Adrenal corticosteroid therapy in far-advanced cancer. Geriatrics. 1972;27:131-41.

12. Oster MH, Enders SR, Samuels SJ, et al. Megestrol acetate in patients with AIDS and cachexia. Ann Int Med. 1994;121:400-8.

13. Gebbia V, Testa A, Gebbia N. Prospective randomised trial of two dose levels of megestrol acetate in the management of anorexia-cachexia syndrome in patients with metastatic cancer. Br J Cancer. 1996;73:1576-80.

14. Loprinzi CL, Schaid DJ, Dose AM, Burnham NL, Jens. Body-composition changes in patients who gain weight while receiving megestrol acetate. J Clin Oncol. 1993;11:152-4.

15. Loprinzi CL, Ellison NM, Schaid DJ, et al. Controlled trial of megestrol acetate for the treatment of cancer anorexia and cachexia. J Natl Cancer Institute. 1990;July 4; 82:1127-32.

16. Van Roenen J, Cleelan C, Gonin R, Hatfield A, Panya K. Physician attitudes and practice in cancer pain management: a survey from the Eastern Cooperative Oncology Group. Ann Intern Med. 1993;119:121-6.

17. Pimentel G, Santos E, Arastu M, Cowan JA. Hyperglycemia in an AIDS patient taking megestrol. Hosp Pract. 1996;31:27-8.

18. Nelson K, Walsh D, Deeter P, Sheehan F. A phase II study of delta-9-tetrahydrocannabinol for appetite stimulation in cancer associated anorexia. J Palliat Care. 1994;10:14-8.

19. Goldberg RM, Loprinzi CL, Mailliard JA, O'Fallon J. Pentoxifylline for treatment of cancer anorexia and cachexia? A randomized, double-blind, placebo-controlled trial. J Clin Oncol. 1995;13:2856-9.

20. Kardinal CG, Loprinzi CL, Schaid DJ, et al. A controlled trial of cyproheptadine in cancer patients with anorexia and/or cachexia. Cancer. 1990;65:2647-62.

21. Chelbowski RT, Bulcavage L, Grosvenor M, et al. Hydrazine sulfate influence on nurtritional status and survival in non-small-cell lung cancer. J Clin Oncol. 1990;8:9-15.

22. Chlebowski RT, Bulcavage L, Grosvernor M, et al. Hydrazine sulfate in cancer patients with weight loss: A placebo-controlled clinical experience. Cancer. 1987;59:406-10.

23. Ackermann M, Kirchner H, Atzpodien J. Low dose megestrol acetate can abrogate cachexia in advanced tumor patients receiving systemic interferon-alfa and/or interleukin-2 based antineoplastic therapy. Anticancer Drugs. 1993;4:585-7.

24. Walsh T. Low-dose megestrol acetate for appetite stimulation. J Pain Sympt Manage. 1995;10:182-3.

Anxiety in Palliative Care Patients

Kenneth C. Jackson II

Arthur G. Lipman

SUMMARY. Anxiety is a common response to life limiting disease, but it can be pathological. Several different disorders are classified as anxiety and therapy for them varies. Potential underlying etiologies and presentations anxiety are discussed. Non-pharmacological therapies and drug therapy for anxiety in palliative care are described. Evaluation instruments that have been used for this symptom are described. Some open research questions are listed. Evidence tables and drug therapy tables which include drug costs are presented. *[Article copies available for a fee from The Haworth Document Delivery Service: 1-800-342-9678. E-mail address: getinfo@haworthpressinc.com <Website: http://www.haworthpressinc.com>]*

KEYWORDS. Anxiety, depression, adjustment disorders, palliative care, terminal care, dying, supportive care, drug therapy, non-pharmacological therapy, etiology, evidence, costs, algorithm, relaxation, muscle, cognitive reframing, distraction, behavioral, benzodiazepines, alprazolam, lorazepam, diazepam, midazolam, chlorpromazine, methotrimeprazine, thioridazine, hydroxyzine, buspirone, propofol, beta blockers, systematic review

Kenneth C. Jackson II, PharmD, is Manager of Clinical Pharmacy Services, St. Dominic-Jackson Memorial Hospital; and Clinical Assistant Professor, University of Mississippi School of Pharmacy, Jackson, MS.

Arthur G. Lipman, PharmD, is Professor, College of Pharmacy; Director of Clinical Pharmacology, Pain Management Center, University Hospitals and Clinics; Pain Medicine and Palliative Care Advisory Group, Huntsman Cancer Center; University of Utah Health Sciences Center, Salt Lake City, UT.

Address correspondence to: Arthur G. Lipman, PharmD, College of Pharmacy and Pain Management Center, 30 S 2000 E RM 258, University of Utah Health Sciences Center, Salt Lake City, UT 84112-5820 (E-mail: alipman@pharm.utah.edu).

[Haworth co-indexing entry note]: "Anxiety in Palliative Care Patients." Jackson, Kenneth C. II, and Arthur G. Lipman. Co-published simultaneously in *Journal of Pharmaceutical Care in Pain & Symptom Control* (Pharmaceutical Products Press, an imprint of The Haworth Press, Inc.) Vol. 7, No. 4, 1999, pp. 23-35, and: *Evidence Based Symptom Control in Palliative Care: Systematic Reviews and Validated Clinical Practice Guidelines for 15 Common Problems in Patients with Life Limiting Disease* (ed: Arthur G. Lipman, Kenneth C. Jackson II, and Linda S. Tyler) Pharmaceutical Products Press, an imprint of The Haworth Press, Inc., 2000, pp. 23-35. Single or multiple copies of this article are available for a fee from The Haworth Document Delivery Service [1-800-342-9678, 9:00 a.m. - 5:00 p.m. (EST). E-mail address: getinfo@haworthpressinc.com].

Algorithm for Managing Anxiety

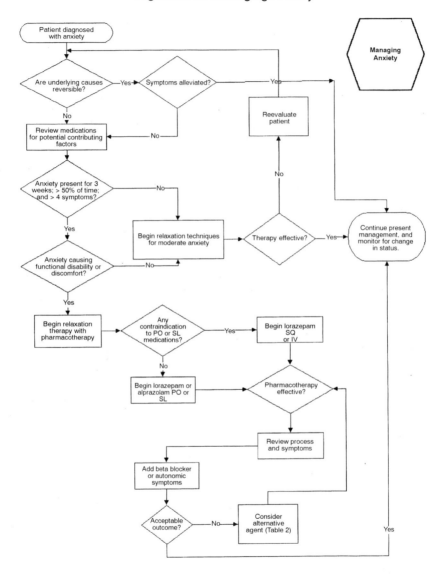

Many patients with life threatening diseases understandably experience anxiety. Anxiety is experienced at some time by most persons, and can be a natural response to the dying process. It becomes problematic when the anxiety is greater than would be construed as a normal response to illness, based on intensity, duration, or dysfunction. Such anxiety is classified as pathological.[1] Impending death may not be the most frequent source of anxiety in cancer patients who may have a range of concerns causing anxiety.[2] These may include adequate pain control, isolation from loved ones, and the needs of their surviving family members. Clinicians' willingness to discuss such issues often lessen anxiety.

Adjustment disorders, obsessive-compulsive disorders, phobias, panic disorders, post-traumatic stress disorder, and generalized anxiety disorders all may be classified as anxiety disorders. The American Psychiatric Association Diagnosis and Statistical manuals, 4th edition (DSM-IV) further clarifies this.

Anxiety may be precipitated by other underlying medical conditions including rheumatoid arthritis and thyroid disorders. Effective management of these underlying causes of anxiety should be a primary goal for palliative care clinicians. Potential causes of anxiety in terminally ill patients include the following.[1,3-8]

POTENTIAL UNDERLYING ETIOLOGIES OF ANXIETY

- cardiac (angina pectoris, arrhythmia's, CHF, MI, valvular disease)
- encephalopathy (infectious, tumors)
- impending cardiac or respiratory arrest
- inadequately controlled pain
- medications
- metabolic (dehydration, hyperkalemia, hyper/hypocalcemia, hypoglycemia, hyponatremia)
- peptic ulcer disease
- psychiatric (depression, delirium)
- respiratory (asthma, COPD, dyspnea, hypoxia, pneumothorax, pulmonary embolism)
- substance withdrawal (alcohol, anticonvulsants, benzodiazepines, clonidine, nicotine, opioids)
- therapy (chemotherapy, radiation)
- tumor related (paraneoplastic syndromes)

Stiefel and Razavi has suggested that anxiety in cancer patients can be classified into four categories: situational anxiety, psychiatric anxiety, organic anxiety, and existential anxiety.[2] Viewing anxiety in this context may allow clinicians to better understand how individuals react to terminal disease. Physiological disturbances may induce organic anxiety. Interdisciplinary care by clergy, nurses, pharmacists, physicians, psychologists, social workers, and volunteers allows the team to better provide for the physical, psychosocial, and spiritual well being of the patient.

The manner in which anxiety presents can provide information useful in defining treatment. Patients with pre-existing anxiety disorders may experience exacerbation or re-activation of a previously controlled anxiety disorder.[5] Patients with pre-existing anxiety should be screened for re-activation of their disease.

Presentation of anxiety can include both psychological and somatic symptoms including apprehension, autonomic hyperactivity, diarrhea, diaphoresis, dyspnea, fear, insomnia nervousness, tremulousness, palpitations, parathesias, uncontrolled worry, and vigilance.[1,4,5,7,9] Physical symptoms are often the first indication of anxiety.[7] When such symptoms present, clinicians should investigate for less obvious psychiatric symptoms of anxiety.

Effective anxiolysis requires that underlying causes be addressed. Many medications have been implicated as causes of anxiety. A thorough review of a patient's medication history is warranted when anxiety is known or suspected. Some medications produce symptoms that can be confused with anxiety, e.g., drug-induced akathisia or motor restlessness. Drugs associated with this type of organic anxiety include chlorpromazine, haloperidol, methotrimeprazine (no longer available in the U.S.), metoclopramide, and prochloperazine.[2,5,9] When questioned, patients taking these medications often are found to be free of the psychological aspects of anxiety.[9] In such cases, cessation of the offending agent should terminate the motor restlessness.

Withdrawal from some drugs can also precipitate anxiety. Alcohol, anticonvulsants, benzodiazepines, clonidine, corticosteroids, nicotine, opioids, and sedative-hypnotics are all known to produce anxiety in withdrawal states.[1,2,5,8]

MEDICATIONS ASSOCIATED
WITH ANXIETY SYMPTOMS[1-7,9-11]

albuterol	amantadine	amphetamine
baclofen	caffeine	chlorpromazine
ciprofloxacin	CMVIG	cocaine
corticosteroids	cycloserine	danazol
dapsone	diethylpropion	digitalis
dopamine	dronabinol	ephedrine
epinephrine	ethanol	fenfluramine
flumazenil	fluoxetine	haloperidol
interferon	isoproterenol	levamisole
methotrimeprazine	methylphenidate	metoclopramide
naphazoline	omeprazole	opioids
oxymetazoline	phenylephrine	phenylpropanolamine
prochloperazine	progestins	pseudoephedrine
sertaline	theophylline	thyroid preparations
traizolam	vigabatrin	

Non-Pharmacological Treatments

While many clinicians use pharmacotherapy as the primary treatment for anxiety, non-drug approaches can be important. Included in these techniques are cognitive reframing, distraction, and progressive muscle relaxation.[1] These behavioral techniques assist patients by enabling them to become educated, correct misconceptions, and reassure them about their situation.[3] Progressive muscle relaxation has been shown to be effective in the management of anxiety symptoms in a randomized clinical trial.[12]

Sources of anxiety should also be reviewed when selecting treatment. Patients suffering from existential anxiety may be better served if they are able to communicate their concerns to a member of the clergy or a counselor. Similarly, patients with financial or legal concerns may benefit from the advice of appropriate professionals. Some may view these as common sense measures, but for many patients these types of concerns (financial, legal, spiritual, etc.) can play a significant role in the pathogenesis of their anxiety state.

Pharmacotherapy

Deciding to use medications in the treatment of anxiety involves a number of factors. As with any form of therapy, benefits and risks from therapy must be weighed. Considerations to the patient's safety and well being must take precedence over other concerns. Maguire and colleagues have stated that patients with moderate anxiety can benefit from non-pharmacological, supportive measures alone.[9] How to determine which patients will best be managed by behavioral techniques alone has not been well defined. Clinicians should consider whether anxiety is interfering with the patient's psychological or physical health. If this is the case, pharmacotherapy should be considered. Whenever possible, psychological interventions should be pursued in addition to drug therapy.

Short-acting benzodiazepines are considered by most authors to be agents of choice for anxiety in terminally ill patients.[1-7,9,13] Alprazolam is the only drug in this class to be studied in clinical trials with terminally ill patients.[12-14]

Holland and colleagues conducted a randomized clinical trial in cancer patients using alprazolam 0.5 mg PO TID for 10 days versus progressive muscle relaxation.[12] Both treatments produced significant improvement in anxiety scores. The alprazolam recipients had a statistically significant greater improvement in anxiety scores, but this appeared to be of marginal clinical significance. This trial only lasted 10 days and dose escalation was not attempted beyond 1.5 mg per day. The authors noted that in their experience these patients respond to lower dosages of alprazolam than physically healthy adults.

Alprazolam also was studied in a randomized, double blind, placebo-controlled trial over a 4-week period.[13] Patients' doses were progressively increased to 4 mg per day during the first week. The average dose of alprazolam received was 1.2 mg per day. Both placebo and drug were shown to effectively reduce anxiety. Three patients in the placebo group with a history of anxiety disorder experienced a worsening of their symptoms. The authors speculate that alprazolam may have a role in treating patients who have a history of anxiety. As with the study by Holland et al.,[12] this study used relatively low daily doses of alprazolam.

Fernandez et al. evaluated alprazolam in 39 patients for its analgesic effect in chronic, organic pain of malignant origin.[14] Eighty-seven percent of the patients exhibited moderate to marked improvements in their psychiatric disorders which were reported to be depression, adjustment disorders, and anxiety disorders. Only one patient with generalized anxiety disorder did not respond to pharmacotherapy and that patient was found to have an organic cause for his anxiety state. Of note, this study's primary end point was pain management. However, the results are interesting especially when faced with the knowledge that many patients will have pain control as a primary or contributing factor for their anxiety.

The American College of Critical Care Medicine and the Society of Critical Care Medicine have developed guidelines with different benzodiazepines as preferred agents in the management of anxiety in critically ill adult patients.[15] While these guidelines were developed for critically ill patients, they may prove useful in palliative care. The guidelines state that either midazolam or propofol should be used as the preferred agent for the short-term treatment of anxiety in this patient population. The authors define short term as less than 24 hours. The guideline also lists lorazepam as the preferred agent for the prolonged treatment of anxiety in the critically ill population. Because these guidelines were developed for hospitalized patients, they may be difficult to extrapolate to palliative care patients receiving care at home.

While benzodiazepines are considered the mainstay of therapy, the review literature lists other agents as having benefit in palliative care. Antidepressants, buspirone, chlorpromazine, haloperidol, hydroxyzine, methotrimeprazine (no longer available in the U.S.), and thioridazine have all been noted to have a role in treating anxiety in this specific patient population.[2-5,7,9] The evidence based palliative care literature has no reference to these agents. However, there are instances in which clinicians may choose to explore the use of these medications. These non-benzodiazepine agents may be considered for patients refractory to benzodiazepine therapy, or who have contraindications to their use. Roth and Breitbart assert that benzodiazepines should be used cautiously or avoided in patients with respiratory compromise.[5] They also state that hydroxyzine, chlorpromazine, and thioridazine can be used safely and effectively without depressing central respiratory function.

The non-benzodiazepine agents may prove to be a better choice in patients with other psychiatric conditions such as organic psychoses or depression.[4,5,7] Although alprazolam may be effective in depression, the other benzodiazepines have not shown efficacy for this indication.[16] Buspirone requires 5 to10 days for initial response in anxiety.[7] Maximum benefit from buspirone may not be seen for 4-6 weeks.[10]

The usefulness of buspirone in treating anxiety in patients with a short life expectancy is limited by this time to effectiveness.

CONCLUSION

Currently there is limited evidence from clinical trials on the role of anxiolytic medications for use in terminally ill patients. Most available literature is anecdotal. What evidence is available indicates that alprazolam, preferably in conjunction with behavioral techniques, is effective in the management of anxiety in cancer patients. There appears to be a consensus in the review literature that lorazepam has a role in palliative care. Additionally, there is support for the use of neuroleptic medications to manage organically-induced anxiety states. The role of atypical antipsychotics, e.g., olanzapine, respiridone, has not been established. When no contraindication exists, drug therapy should be initiated with either alprazolam or lorazepam. Other medications may prove to be useful agents, but at this time they should be reserved for second line of therapy.

SOME OPEN RESEARCH QUESTIONS

- Are higher dosages of alprazolam indicated in terminally ill patients?
- How do other psychiatric disease states impact pharmacotherapy of anxiety? Should subset analysis occur to determine type of therapy most beneficial?
- Should non-pharmacological strategies receive a higher priority in the management of patients?
- Would alprazolam be effective in anxious and depressed terminally ill patients?
- How should the expected life expectancy affect the antianxiety drug therapy of choice?
- Do organic/functional etiologies predict different therapeutic responses from interventions?
- What role do midazolam and propofol have in palliative care?
- Are the newer atypical antipsychotic agents olanzapine, respiridone effective in managing anxiety in palliative care?

TABLE 1. Drug Therapy for Managing Anxiety in Palliative Care Evidence Table–Alprazolam (Xanax)

Reference	Study Design	n	Intervention	Results	Level of Evidence	Comments
Fernandez (1987)[12]	Descriptive	39	Alprazolam used for analgesic effect. Patients selected if had underlying mood or anxiety disorder. Effective doses ranged from 1.5-4.0 mg/day.	87% showed moderate to marked improvement in their psychiatric disorder, as rated by The Clinical Global Judgement Scale. One patient with generalized anxiety disorder did not respond to alprazolam.	V	Main focus of the article is on the use of alprazolam as an adjunct in pain management.
Wald (1993)[13]	Randomized Double-blind Placebo controlled	36	Starting alprazolam dose of 0.5 mg/day, increased to 4 mg/day over the the first week. Minor adjustments made if anxiety increased or side effects developed.	Equal efficacy noted with both placebo and active treatment (p = .0001). However, alprazolam did decrease scores in 6 of 6 patients with a history of anxiety disorder. Placebo demonstrated a decrease in 3 of 6 patients with a history of an anxiety disorder.	II	Average alprazolam dose was 1.2 mg/day. Higher doses may have altered the outcome.
Holland (1991)[14]	Randomized	147	Alprazolam arm: given 0.5 mg tid for 10 days, then tapered off drug over 3 days. Relaxation arm: Initial training with behavioral psychologist, then used tape at home tid for 10 days.	Both treatments improved anxiety scores (p < .001 Hamilton Anxiety Rating Scale, Affects Balance Scale, Symptoms Checklist-90), with the drug arm exhibiting a marginally better decrease in anxiety scores (p = .04 for Hamilton Anxiety Rating Scale and p = .02 for Affects Balance Scale).	II	Unblinded study. Dose limited to 0.5 mg tid.

Key to Level of evidence classification:

Level I   Randomized trials with low false-positive (alpha) and low false-negative (beta errors); high power
Level II   Randomized trials with high false-positive (alpha) and/or high false-negative (beta errors); low power
Level III Nonrandomized concurrent cohort comparisons between contemporaneous patients who did and did not receive a given intervention
Level IV Nonrandomized historical cohort comparisons between current patients who receive the intervention and patients (from the same institution or from the literature) who did not
Level V   Case series without control subjects

TABLE 2. Anxiolytic Medications for Use in the Terminally Ill Drug Regimens of Choice[1,3-7,9-16]

Drug	Routes	Dose	AWP per Day of Therapy#		Other
alprazolam (Xanax)	PO, SL[17,18]	Initial: mg tid Maintenance: Up to 4 mg/day Procedural anxiety: 0.5 mg PO 30-60 minutes prior to procedure	0.25 mg PO tid 1 mg PO qid	$ 0.15/day $ 0.32/day	Doses as high as 10 mg/day may be needed for patients with panic disorder. Metabolism impaired by fluoxetine, fluvoxamine, nefazodone Peak oral serum levels sooner than lorazepam
lorazepam (Ativan)	PO, SL[19,20], IM, IV	Initial: mg PO tid Maintenance: 2-10 mg PO/daily Procedural anxiety: 2-4 mg IV 15 minutes prior to procedure	0.5 mg PO tid 2 mg PO qid 2 mg IM/IV qid	$ 0.05/day $ 0.09/day $ 2.15/day	Benefits of multiple routes of administration Preferred in patients with hepatic dysfunction Preferred agent for prolonged treatment of anxiety of critically ill adults
hydroxyzine (Vistaril)	PO, IM	Initial: 10 mg PO qid Maintenance: 10-50 mg PO Q4-6 hours	10 mg PO qid 50 mg IM Q6H	$ 0.09/day $ 2.88/day	antihistamine IV use associated with hemolysis SC and Intra-arterial use associated with tissue necrosis potentiates analgesic effects of morphine
diazepam (Valium)	PO, IV, PR	Initial: 5 mg PO bid Maintenance: 5-10 mg PO bid-qid	5 mg PO bid 5 mg IV bid	$ 0.03/day $ 6.85/day	Benefit of rectal administration Long half-life (> 24 hrs)
chlorpromazine (Thorazine)	PO, PR, IM, IV	Initial: 10-25 mg PO tid Maintenance: 2.5-50 mg PO Q4-12 hours	25 mg PO tid 25 mg PR tid 25 mg IV tid 50 mg PO tid	$ 0.18/day $ 8.87/day $21.77 $ 0.20/day	Monitor for extrapyramidal effects Anticholinergic properties may exacerbate delirium Watch for hypotension with IM or IV use

Drug	Route	Dosing	Dose / Cost[#]	Comments
thioridazine (Mellaril)	PO	Initial: 10 mg PO tid Maintenance: 10-75 mg PO tid-qid	50 mg PO tid $ 0.16/day	Geriatric dose is 20-25% of dose used in younger adults Monitor for extrapyramidal effects Anticholinergic properties may exacerbate delirium
buspirone (Buspar)	PO	Initial: 5 mg tid Maintenance: 10-20 mg tid	5 mg PO tid $ 1.80/day 10 mg PO tid $ 3.11/day	Usefulness limited by delayed onset of action (may have role in chronic therapy) Doses of 60 mg/day associated with dysphoria No cross tolerance with benzodiazepines May increase haloperidol serum levels Avoid use with MAO Inhibitors (possible hypertension)
methotrimeprazine (Levoprome) (no longer available in the U.S.)	SQ, IM	Initial: 10 mg IM Q 8 hours Maintenance: 10-20 mg IM or SQ Q4-8 hours	10 mg IM Q8H $27.23/day	Phenothiazine Available only in parenteral form (USA) Useful for sedative properties Monitor for hypertension Anticholinergic properties may exacerbate delirium SQ not recommended due to local irritation
midazolam (Versed)	SQ, IV	Initial: .03 mg/kg Maintenance: .03 mg/kg/hr Titrate to clinical response	10 mg IV/SQ per day $19.07/day	Doses of 2-10 mg/day normally seen Doses of 30-60 mg/day have been reported Rapid onset Short duration of action Tolerated subcutaneously
propofol (Diprivan)	IV	Initial: 0.5 mg/kg/hr Maintenance: 0.5-3.0 mg/kg/hr Titrate to clinical response	5 mg IV per hour $ 7.71/day 70 mg IV per hour $107.92/day	Dose will vary by clinical response Requires IV access Requires continuous administration Rapid onset Short duration of action Easily contaminated

Average Wholesale Price, 1999 (cost to pharmacy)

REFERENCES

1. Noyes R, Holt CS, Massie MJ. Anxiety disorders. In: Holland JC, ed. Psychooncology. New York: Oxford University Press; 1998:548-563.

2. Stiefel F, Razavi D. Common psychiatric disorders in cancer patients II. Anxiety and acute confusional states. Support Care Cancer. 1994;2:233-237.

3. Bluestine S, Lesko L. Psychotropic medications in oncology and in AIDS patients. Adv Psychosom Med. 1994;21:107-137.

4. Breitbart W, Jacobsen PB. Psychiatric symptom management in terminal care. Clin Geriatr Med. 1996;12:329-347.

5. Roth AJ, Breitbart W. Psychiatric emergencies in terminally ill cancer patients. Pain and Palliat Care. 1996;10:235-259.

6. Payne DK, Massie MJ. Depression and anxiety. In: Berger AM, Portenoy RK, Weissman DE, eds. Principles and Practice of Supportive Oncology. Philadelphia, PA: Lippincott-Raven Publishers; 1998:497-511.

7. Breitbart W, Passik SD. Psychiatric aspects of palliative care. In: Doyle D, Hanks GWC, Macdonald N, eds. Oxford Textbook of Palliative Medicine. New York: Oxford University Press; 1993:609-626.

8. Knoben JE, Anderson PO. Handbook of Clinical Drug Data. 8 ed. Stamford, CT: Appleton and Lange; 1997.

9. Maguire P, Faulkner A, Regnard C. Managing the anxious patient with advancing disease–a flow diagram. Palliative Medicine. 1993;7:239-244.

10. Kirkwood CK, Hayes PE. Anxiety Disorders JT. Anxiety Disorders. In Pharmacotherapy, 3rd edition, Dipiro J. Talbert R, Yee G, et al., eds, Stamford CT. Appleton and Lange, 1997.

11. Lacy C, Armstrong LL, Ingrim N, Lance LL. Drug Information Handbook. 3rd ed: Lexi-comp; 1995.

12. Holland JC, Morrow GR, Schmale A, et al. A randomized clinical trial of alprazolam versus progressive muscle relaxation in cancer patients with anxiety and depressive symptoms. J Clin Oncol. 1991;9:1004-1011.

13. Wald TG, Kathol RG, Noyes R, Carroll BT, Clamon GH. Rapid relief of anxiety in cancer patients with both alprazolam and placebo. Psychosomatics. 1993;34:324-332.

14. Fernandez F, Adams F, Holmes VF. Analgesic effect of alprazolam in patients with chronic, organic pain of malignant origin. J Clin Psychopharmacol. 1987; 7:167-169.

15. Shapiro BA, Warren J, Egol AB, et al. Practice parameters for intravenous analgesia and sedation for adult patients in the intensive care unit: an executive summary. Crit Care Med. 1995;23:1596-1600.

16. Levy MH, Catalano RB. Control of common physical symptoms other than pain in patients with terminal disease. Seminars in Oncology. 1985;12:411-430.

17. Scavone JM, Greenblatt DJ, Goddard JE, Friedman H, Harmatz JS, Shader RI. The pharmacokinetics and pharmacodynamics of sublingual and oral alprazolam in the post-prandial state. Eur J Clin Pharmacol. 1992;42:439-443.

18. Scavone JM, Greenblatt DJ, Shader RI. Alprazolam kinetics following sublingual and oral administration. J Clin Psychopharmacol. 1987;77:332-334.

19. Spenard J, Caille G, de Montigny C, et al. Placebo-controlled comparative study of the anxiolytic activity and of the pharmacokinetics of oral and sublingual lorazepam in generalized anxiety. Biopharm Drug Dispos. 1988;9:457-464.

20. Enck RE. The last few days. Am J Hosp Palliat Care. 1992;9:11-13.

Bleeding Problems
in Palliative Care Patients

M. Christine Jamjian

SUMMARY. Bleeding problems occur commonly with certain cancers and other degenerative diseases. Causes and supportive care of bleeding and oozing are described. Experience with fibrinolytic inhibitors, topical hemostats, and systemic pharmacotherapy is summarized. Evaluation instruments that have been used for this symptom are described. Some open research questions are listed. A treatment algorithm, evidence tables and drug therapy tables which include drug costs are presented. *[Article copies available for a fee from The Haworth Document Delivery Service: 1-800-342-9678. E-mail address: getinfo@haworthpressinc. com <Website: http://www.haworthpressinc.com>]*

KEYWORDS. Bleeding, oozing, platelets, thrombocytopenia, palliative care, terminal care, dying, supportive care, drug therapy, non-pharmacological therapy, etiology, evidence, costs, algorithm, fibrinolytic inhibitors, topical hemostatic, hemostat, tranexamic acid, aminocaproic acid, cellulose, gelatin, thrombin, collagen, sponge, disseminated intravascular coagulopathy, DIC, coagulation, fibrinolysis, vascular, systematic review

M. Christine Jamjian, PharmD, is Clinical Pharmacist, HIV Clinic, Department of Pharmacy Services, University Hospitals and Clinics, University of Utah, Salt Lake City, UT.

Address correspondence to: Arthur G. Lipman, PharmD, College of Pharmacy and Pain Management Center, 30 S 2000 E RM 258, University of Utah Health Sciences Center, Salt Lake City, UT 84112-5820 (E-mail: alipman@pharm.utah.edu).

[Haworth co-indexing entry note]: "Bleeding Problems in Palliative Care Patients." Jamjian, M. Christine. Co-published simultaneously in *Journal of Pharmaceutical Care in Pain & Symptom Control* (Pharmaceutical Products Press, an imprint of The Haworth Press, Inc.) Vol. 7, No. 4, 1999, pp. 37-46; and: *Evidence Based Symptom Control in Palliative Care: Systematic Reviews and Validated Clinical Practice Guidelines for 15 Common Problems in Patients with Life Limiting Disease* (ed: Arthur G. Lipman, Kenneth C. Jackson II, and Linda S. Tyler) Pharmaceutical Products Press, an imprint of The Haworth Press, Inc., 2000, pp. 37-46. Single or multiple copies of this article are available for a fee from The Haworth Document Delivery Service [1-800-342-9678, 9:00 a.m. - 5:00 p.m. (EST). E-mail address: getinfo@haworthpressinc.com].

37

Algorithm for Management of Oozing/Bleeding

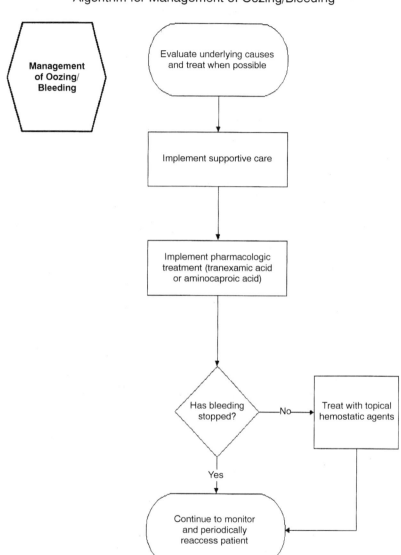

Malignancies and other degenerative diseases can cause hemostatic changes that lead to hematological disturbances. Diagnosis and management of hemorrhage and thrombosis in cancer patients have been studied extensively. However, data are lacking on optimal management of bleeding or oozing from mucosal membranes, specifically as part of a palliative care treatment plan. Table 1 outlines the evidence on managing cancer-associated bleeding or oozing with pharmacological interventions. The following summarizes a treatment strategy for managing these patients and selecting appropriate pharmacologic agents.

EVALUATE THE CAUSES OF BLEEDING AND OOZING

Each patient with oozing should be evaluated, potential causes identified, and contributing factors ascertained. When possible, the underlying cause of the symptoms should be treated. Frequent causes of bleeding that can be treated include:

- Thrombocytopenia
- Platelet dysfunction
- Disseminated intravascular coagulation
- Coagulation protein defects
- Primary fibrinolysis
- Vascular defects

IMPLEMENT SUPPORTIVE CARE

Non-pharmacological measures can be implemented to treat bleeding. These include:

- Apply pressure over the wound
- Protect bleeding area from trauma
- Remove infected granulation tissue
- Keep area clean
- Suture tissues for primary closure when possible and support of wound margins

TREAT CANCER-ASSOCIATED BLEEDING OR OOZING PHARMACOLOGICALLY

Several pharmacologic agents have been evaluated to manage bleeding in cancer patients. These are summarized in Tables 2 and 3.

TABLE 1. Drug Therapy for Managing Bleeding and Oozing in Palliative Care Evidence Table

Reference	Study Design	n	Intervention	Results	Level of Evidence
Tranexamic Acid (Cyklokapron) and Aminocaproic Acid (Amicar)					
Dean (1997)[1]	Descriptive	16	Patients with tumor-associated bleeding or unable to have definitive hemostatic treatment were offered treatment with tranexamic acid or aminocaproic acid depending on the availability of fibrinolytic inhibitor within the treating hospital. Tranexamic acid dose was 1.5 grams as an loading dose, then 1 gram tid. Aminocaproic acid dose was 5 grams as a loading dose, then 1 gram qid. Treatment was continued until 7 days after bleeding has stopped.	15 patients noted improvement of bleeding. 14 patients had complete cessation of bleeding. The average time to improvement was 2 days. The average time to bleeding cessation was 4 days.	V
Topical Hemostatic Agent					
Green (1991)[4]	Descriptive	1	Patient with thrombocytopenia and persistent complaint of gingival hemorrhage. INSTAT collagen was applied locally to control bleeding. Patient also received platelets.	Episodes of gingival hemorrhage were controlled adequately with platelet transfusions and topical hemostat.	V
O'Halpin (1984)[5]	Descriptive	48	Patients with acute hemorrhage, patients who required preoperative vascular control, individuals with inoperable lesions, or various unusual lesions had arterial embolization performed during a five year period. The occlusive used were Gelfoam, oxidized cellulose, isobutyl-2-cyanoacrylate mixed with Myodii, Gianturco wire coils and lyophilized dura mater.	The procedure was successful in controlling hemorrhage(14/15), managing inoperable lesions (10/10), and treating unusual lesions (7/7). Patients who required pre-operative vascular control did not benefit from arterial embolization (4/16)	V
Griska (1981)[6]	Descriptive	1	Patient with pharyngeal carcinoma experienced massive bleeding from the posterior pharyngeal wall. Ligation of external carotid arteries was impossible. Embolization was recommended. Gelfoam was used for bilateral embolization the superior thyroid, ascending pharyngeal, lingual, facial, and internal maxillary branches of the external carotid arteries.	Bleeding was completely controlled. No complications occurred. Packing was removed with no further complications. Patient died several week later from bleeding by tumor outside area previously embolized.	V

Russinovich (1980)[8]	Descriptive	1	Patient with persistent bleeding after a transurethral prostatic resection had successful transcatheter hypogastric arterial embolization with Gelfoam.	Patient experienced prompt cessation of bleeding	V
Masuda (1989)[7]	Descriptive	2	Patient with carcinoma of the tongue presented with hemorrhage from his ulcerated tongue. Gauze packing with bosmin was ineffective in controlling the bleeding. Transcatheter embolization with Gelfoam was performed. Patient with tongue carcinoma was also treated with embolization to stop hemorrhage from that area.	Bleeding from the tongue stopped completely. Patients died after two months and autopsy results revealed necrosis of the embolized lingual artery. Bleeding completely stopped.	V

Key to Level of Evidence Classification:

Level I   Randomized trials with low false-positive (alpha) and low false-negative (beta errors); high power
Level II   Randomized trials with high false-positive (alpha) and/or high false-negative (beta errors); low power
Level III   Non-randomized concurrent cohort comparisons between contemporaneous patients who did and did not receive a given intervention
Level IV   Non-randomized historical cohort comparisons between current patients who did receive the intervention and patients (from the same institution or from the literature) who did not
Level V   Case series without control subjects

TABLE 2. Drug Therapy for Managing Bleeding in the Cancer Patient

Drug Therapy	Indications for Use	Dosing Regimen	AWP per Day of Therapy#
aminocaproic Acid (Amicar) (500 mg tablets)	One case report supports its use in patients with tumor associated bleeding unable to receive definitive hemostatic treatment.	5 grams po × 1 dose then 1 gram po qid	$12.54/5 grams $10.00/day
tranexamic Acid (Cyklokapron) (500 mg tablets)	One case report supports its use in patients with tumor associated bleeding unable to receive definitive hemostatic treatment.	1.5 grams po × 1 dose then 1 gram po tid	$9.45/1.5 grams $18.90/day

Average Wholesale Price, 1999 (cost to pharmacy)

TABLE 3. Topical Hemostatic Agents for the Management of Bleeding in the Cancer Patient

Hemostatic Agent (Proprietary Names)	Indications for Use	Method of Usage	Precautions	AWP
thrombin (Thrombostat, Thrombogen)	It might be useful in hard to reach areas and also under the sternum. It acts by clotting the fibrinogen of the blood directly. This agent is useless in the absence of fibrinogen.	1. Surface of oozing area should be sponged free of blood. 2. Allow mixture with blood as soon as it reaches the surface.	Since it is an antigenic substance, allergic reaction can occur.	$18.56-$65.63 per vial
absorbable gelatin sponge (Gelfoam)	Gelatin sponge can be used dry or moistened with thrombin solution or saline. It also can be used as an occlusive agent during transcatheter embolization.	1. Cut the sheet to size. 2. Apply to the bleeding site. 3. A cotton pledget or gauze should be placed on the sponge. 4. Before removal of the cotton pledget or sponge, they should be moistened with saline to prevent dislodging the clot.	Infection is a concern with absorbable gelatin sponge. Since sponge absorbs blood, increased pressure can be exerted in confined areas. It is contraindicated in the presence of infection, biliary drainage, or intestinal spillage.	$30/sponge
microfibrillar collagen hemostat (MCH) (Avitene)	MCH is a good choice to control oozing from vascular anastomotic sites. MCH acts by providing a surface of interstices for aggregation of platelets where platelets can undergo their release action.	1. Exert pressure on targeted area 2. Apply MCH. 3. Apply further pressure by using a sponge. 4. After 5 to 10 minutes, excess should be removed.	Infection can occur with MCH. Allergic reactions can also occur because it is a bovine product. MCH can be washed by brisk bleeding.	$93.23 per g
absorbable collagen sheet hemostat (Instat)	Acts by allowing platelets to aggregate and release coagulation factors which with plasma factors lead to fibrin and clot formation.	Apply to bleeding site with pressure.	Adhesion formation, allergic reactions, and foreign body reactions are a concern with these products.	$50-$200 per pad
absorbable collagen sponge (Helistat)	Acts by providing a surface of interstices for aggregation of platelets where platelets can undergo their release action.	Apply to bleeding site with pressure.	It can cause allergic reactions. It should not be used in skin closure.	
Oxidized cellulose (Oxycel) oxidized regenerated cellulose (Surgicel, Nu-Knit)	These agents do not affect the clotting mechanism. They absorb blood and form a gelatinous mass that leads to clot formation. The mass absorbs blood and as such exert pressure. Oxycel can interfere with epithelialization; Surgicel does not. All are bactericidal due to low pH.	Apply dry. Remove after clot formation. Use only amount needed.	These agents should be removed from confined areas due to ability to exert pressure on surrounding tissues. They should not be used to wrap around vascular anastomotic sites. They should not be implanted in bone defects.	$34.50-$79.50 per sheet (Oxycel) $7-$30 persheet (Surgicel and Nu-Knit)

43

Fibrinolytic Inhibitors

Tranexamic acid and aminocaproic acid are antifibrinolytic agents that prevent the lysis of fibrin clots by inhibiting plasmin activation. Both drugs are well absorbed from the gastrointestinal tract. Forty percent of tranexamic acid is excreted in the urine within 24 hours whereas 75% of aminocaproic acid is eliminated within 12 hours. Dose adjustments are required when these drugs are used in patients with renal insufficiency. Nausea, vomiting, and diarrhea are the most common adverse events noted with these drugs.

An open label, non-randomized study[1] evaluated the effectiveness of tranexamic acid and aminocaproic acid in the palliative treatment of tumor-associated bleeding. Sixteen patients with tumor associated bleeding were included in the study. Patients received either tranexamic acid or aminocaproic acid depending on which agent was available in the institution. Improvement of bleeding was observed in 15 of the patients while complete cessation was noted in 14 patients. The average time period to improvement was two days while it took an average of four days for complete bleeding cessation. Recurrence of bleeding occurred in 3 patients.

Topical Hemostatic Agents

Microfibrillar collagen hemostat (Avitene, others), collagen absorbable hemostat (INSTAT), topical thrombin sponges (Gelfoam, Actifoam, Helistat), and oxidized regenerated cellulose (Surgicel) can all be used to control bleeding.[2] None of these agents replaces systemic interventions; they are complimentary therapies. All of these products have been used extensively to manage of bleeding following surgical procedures. An *in vitro* analysis of topical hemostatic agents showed collagen-based agents to be more effective in inducing platelet aggregation and secretion than gelatin or oxidized regenerated cellulose based agents.[3] One case report described the use of an absorbable collagen sheet (INSTAT) hemostat successfully in the management of gingival hemorrhage in a patient with thrombocytopenia.[4] Therapeutic arterial embolization using an absorbable gelatin sponge (Gelfoam), oxidized cellulose, or isobutyl-2-cyoacrylate as occlusive agents was effective in several cases in reducing or halting cancer-related bleeding.[5-8]

Transcatheter embolization can be complicated by the accidental occlusion of a vessel other than the one intended. Further complications encountered with artificial embolization include ischemia, tissue necrosis, and cerebral embolization. The choice of occlusive agent depends on the lesion, the size of the vessel, the indication for embolization, and whether the occlusion is permanent or temporary. Isobutyl-2-cyoacrylate is a permanent occlusive agent that can be placed in the core of a lesion for complete occlusion of medium and large vessels.[5] Gelfoam provides temporary occlusion of medium-sized vessels.

SOME RESEARCH QUESTIONS

1. Which patients would benefit the most from fibrinolytic inhibitor agents?
2. What topical agent is the most useful in managing oozing in the cancer patient?
3. When should therapy be initiated and when should it not be started?
4. Do different topical hemostatic agents vary in usefulness in managing oozing in cancer patients?
5. Are any agents therapeutically interchangeable?
6. Is there a need to study the effectiveness of fibrinolytic inhibitors in a larger sample of cancer patients for the management of oozing?
7. Are there any differences between the topical hemostatic agents when used to control bleeding in terminally ill patients?
8. Are there any differences between aminocaproic acid and tranexamic acid when used to control bleeding in terminally ill patients?
9. What is the optimal dose of aminocaproic acid and tranexamic acid to control bleeding?
10. Do patients with thrombocytopenia have different patient outcomes than patients with normal platelets when fibrinolytic inhibitors and topical hemostatic agents are used? Do other strategies also need to be used for these patients?

REFERENCES

1. Dean A, Tuffin P. Fibrinolytic inhibitors for cancer-associated bleeding problems. J Pain Symptom Manage. 1997;13:20-24.

2. Moak E. Hemostatic agents. Adjuncts to control bleeding. Today's O.R. Nurse. 1991;13:6-10.

3. Wagner W, Pachence J, Ristich J, et al. Comparative *in vitro* analysis of topical hemostatic agents. J Surg Res. 1996;66:100-108.

4. Green J, Durham T. Application of INSTAT hemostat in the control of gingival hemorrhage in the patient with thrombocytopenia. Oral Surg Oral Med Oral Pathol. 1991;71:27-30.

5. O'Halpin D, Legge D, MacErlean D. Therapeutic arterial embolization: Report of five years experience. Clin Radiol. 1984;35:85-93.

6. Griska L, Aghamohamadi A, Marlowe F, et al. Embolization of hemorrhage caused by carcinoma of the pharynx. Head Neck Surg. 1981;3:202-203.

7. Masuda G, Nagamori T, Kawabe R, et al. Utilization of therapeutic embolization in hemorrhage caused by carcinoma of the tongue. J Craniomaxillofac Surg. 1989;17:323-325.

8. Russinovich N, Stauffer A, Griggs P, et al. Transcatheter Gelfoam embolization in intractable prostatic bleeding. Urol Radiol. 1979;1:179-181

Constipation in Palliative Care Patients

M. Christina Beckwith

SUMMARY. Constipation is a common result of advanced disease and drug therapy. It occurs in as many as 50% of advanced cancer patients and 85% of patients taking high dose opioids. Potential causes are described. Prevention and early reversal are important. Nondrug and pharmacological methods of preventing and treating constipation are described. Evaluation instruments that have been used for this symptom are described. Some open research questions are listed. A management algorithm, evidence tables, and drug therapy tables which include drug costs are presented. *[Article copies available for a fee from The Haworth Document Delivery Service: 1-800-342-9678. E-mail address: getinfo@ haworthpressinc.com <Website: http://www.haworthpressinc.com>]*

KEYWORDS. Constipation, bowels, impaction, palliative care, terminal care, dying, opioids, prevention, supportive care, drug therapy, non-pharmacological therapy, etiology, evidence, costs, algorithm, senna, casanthranol, bisacodyl, sorbitol, lactulose, milk of magnesia, sodium phosphate, sodium biphosphate, enemas, minienemas, naloxone, manual evacuation, docusate, glycerin, abdominal, flatulence, bloating, malaise, nausea, systematic review

---

M. Christina Beckwith, PharmD, is Drug Information Specialist, Department of Pharmacy Services, University Hospitals and Clinics, University of Utah, Salt Lake City, UT.

Address correspondence to: Arthur G. Lipman, PharmD, College of Pharmacy and Pain Management Center, 30 S 2000 E RM 258, University of Utah Health Sciences Center, Salt Lake City, UT 84112-5820 (E-mail: alipman@pharm.utah.edu).

[Haworth co-indexing entry note]: "Constipation in Palliative Care Patients." Beckwith, M. Christina. Co-published simultaneously in *Journal of Pharmaceutical Care in Pain & Symptom Control* (Pharmaceutical Products Press, an imprint of The Haworth Press, Inc.) Vol. 7, No. 4, 1999, pp. 47-57; and: *Evidence Based Symptom Control in Palliative Care: Systematic Reviews and Validated Clinical Practice Guidelines for 15 Common Problems in Patients with Life Limiting Disease* (ed: Arthur G. Lipman, Kenneth C. Jackson II, and Linda S. Tyler) Pharmaceutical Products Press, an imprint of The Haworth Press, Inc., 2000, pp. 47-57. Single or multiple copies of this article are available for a fee from The Haworth Document Delivery Service [1-800-342-9678, 9.00 a.m. - 5:00 p.m. (EST). E-mail address: getinfo@haworthpressinc.com].

Algorithm for Managing Constipation

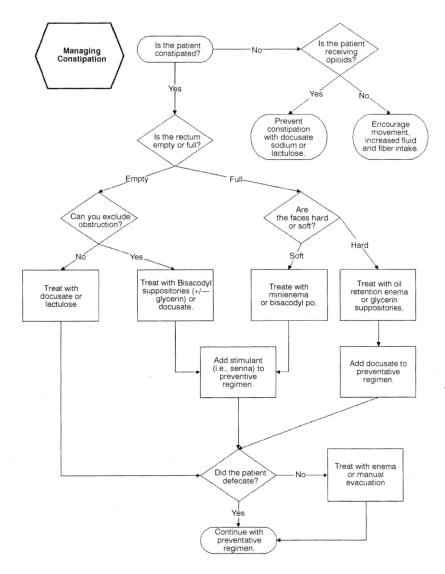

Constipation occurs in approximately half of all patients with advanced cancer[3-5] and in over 85% of patients receiving opioids.[1,3] It also occurs in a large number of patients with advanced disease of many other causes. Several causes and consequences of constipation in palliative care patients have been reported.[1,2] In one case series of cancer patients, constipation was a more frequent cause of severe distress than pain.[6] Few clinical trials have evaluated the efficacy of medications for constipation in palliative care patients. Table 1 summarizes the evidence from available trials for managing constipation with pharmacologic interventions.

EVALUATE THE CAUSES OF CONSTIPATION

Each patient with constipation should be evaluated for potential causes. Constipation is defined as either reduced frequency or increased difficulty of defecation.[7] Frequency of defecation varies widely among individuals, with approximately 95% of the American and British populations defecating between 3 times a day and 3 times a week. Constipation may be associated with abdominal pain, flatulence, and bloating; malaise and nausea.[3]

Both the patient's bowel function history and expectations for bowel movements should be assessed. Rectal and abdominal examinations should be performed to rule out malignant obstruction and fecal impaction.[3] To guide selection of therapy, patient evaluation should determine if the rectum contains feces, whether feces in the rectum are hard or soft, and whether the colon contains feces if the rectum is empty. To assist in future evaluations, it is useful to record any bowel movements, rectal examination findings, and interventions tried.

TREAT THE UNDERLYING CAUSE WHEN POSSIBLE

Whenever possible, the underlying cause of the symptoms should be treated. Frequent treatable causes of constipation include

- anorexia
- inadequate fluid intake
- inadequate dietary fiber intake

- decreased activity
- weakness
- decreased abdominal muscle tone
- inconvenient toilet access and poor posture
- hypothyroidism
- depression
- hypercalcemia
- hypokalemia
- intestinal obstruction by tumor in the bowel wall or compressing the bowel from the pelvis or abdomen

IMPLEMENT SUPPORTIVE THERAPY

Non-pharmacologic measures which can be implemented to treat constipation include the following.

- discontinue or reduce dosage of constipating medications, including:

   opioid analgesics, nonsteroidal anti-inflammatory agents, tricyclic antidepressants, phenothiazines, haloperidol, antiparkinsonian agents, diuretics, iron supplements, and aluminum-containing antacids. This strategy may not be appropriate for all palliative care patients.
- increase fluid intake with a goal intake of 8 glasses daily, providing a variety of fluids.
- increase dietary fiber.
- increase activity. Even minimal exercise may be helpful, such as moving from bed to a chair, or moving around in the bed.
- manual removal of fecal impaction, if present.
- abdominal massage.
- increase accessibility and privacy of toilet facilities.
- establish a regular bowel routine. Since the strongest propulsive contractions occur after breakfast, provide the patient with privacy and access to the toilet at this time every day.

MANAGE CONSTIPATION PHARMACOLOGICALLY

The goal of pharmacologic therapy is to prevent constipation and, failing that, to treat it. Although controlled clinical trials are lacking in

TABLE 1. Drug Therapy for Managing Constipation in Palliative Care Evidence Tables

Reference	Study Design	n	Intervention	Results	Level of Evidence	Comments
Lactulose						
Crowther (1978)[11]	Descriptive	46	Terminally ill patients received oral lactulose 20 mL daily for 21 days, increasing dose as needed for patient comfort and satisfaction. Patients treated with senna, suppositories, enemas, or manual evacuation as necessary. Some patients on opiates although percentage not reported.	Irritant laxatives (i.e., senna) required in 5 of 31 evaluable patients, glycerin suppositories in 14/31 patients, enemas in 7/31 patients, and manual evacuation in 8/31 patients. Of 203 stools passed, 71.5% described as easy to move.	V	Average lactulose dose was 20 mL twice daily. Lactulose resulted in a bowel movement every 2-3 days, despite intensive opiate therapy. Fecal incontinence due to lactulose was rare.
Harris (1977)[12]	Descriptive	8	Vincristine-treated cancer patients received oral lactulose 20 mL 2 time/day upto 25 mL 3 times/day. Did not report whether or not patients receiving opioids.	All patients had a bowel movement within 2 days. Serum electrolytes were unchanged by lactulose therapy.	V	None.
Naloxone (Narcan)						
Sykes (1996)[14]	Phase I: Randomized, double-blind, placebo-controlled	16	Randomized to oral naloxone or placebo. Based on response, patients received daily naloxone dose of 0.5%, 1%, 2%, 5%, 10%, or 20% of daily morphine dose for 1 day.	Of 12 evaluable patients, 2 each received naloxone doses of 0.5%, 1.0%, 2.0%, and 5.0%. Three patients received naloxone dose of 10.0% and one received 20%. No significant change in small bowel transit time (p = 0.43 vs. placebo) or reduction in pain control with naloxone (p = 0.44 vs. placebo).	II	Diarrhea reported in 2 patients receiving naloxone doses of 20% of daily morphine dose.
	Phase II: Open, dose-ranging	10	Patients given daily oral naloxone doses of 20%, 40%, or 80% of daily morphine dose. Cancer patients receiving regular oral opioids for pain control. Allowed to take other laxatives besides lactulose. Total daily dose of naloxone or placebo divided and given every 4 hours. Small bowel transit time measured with lactulose/hydrogen test.	Naloxone dose of ≥20% had a laxative effect. Two generalized withdrawal reactions occurred.	V	Patients received lactulose 15 mL orally for testing small bowel transit time; may have affected study results.

TABLE 1 (continued)

Reference	Study Design	n	Intervention	Results	Level of Evidence	Comments
Sorbitol						
Lederle et al. (1990)[9]	Randomized, double-blind, crossover	30	Elderly men with chronic constipation received lactulose and sorbitol up to 60 mL daily for 4 weeks in random order with a 2 week washout period. Other laxatives not allowed except bulk forming agents. Opioids not allowed	No difference between sorbitol and lactulose in ave. number of bowel movements (6.71 vs. 7.02, p > 0.3), ave. days/week with movements (5.23 vs. 5.31, p > 0.3), or percent "normal" movements (59.8 vs. 66.6, p > 0.3)		
Senna, Sennosoids, Standardized Senna Concentrate (Senokot)						
Agra (1998)[13]	Randomized Open	91	Terminally ill patients received either oral lactulose 15 mL (10 g) daily or senna 0.4 mL (12 mg) for 27 days. Doses were increased if no evacuation noted in 3 days. Maximum doses were 1.6 mL (48 mg) of senna and 60 mL (40 g) of lactulose.	No difference in efficacy or toxicity noted between laxatives.	I	Authors recommend the use of senna based on favorable toxicity profile and cost advantage.
Sykes (1996)[14]	Phase I: Randomized, double-blind, placebo-controlled	16	Randomized to oral naloxone or placebo. Based on response, patients received daily naloxone dose of 0.5%, 1%, 2%, 5%, 10%, or 20% of daily morphine dose for 1 day. Patients given daily oral naloxone doses of 20%, 40%, or 80% of daily morphine dose.	Of 12 evaluable patients, 2 each received naloxone doses of 0.5%, 1.0%, 2.0%, and 5.0%. Three patients received naloxone dose of 10.0% and one received 20%. No significant change in small bowel transit time (p = 0.43 vs. placebo) or reduction in pain control with naloxone (p = 0.44 vs. placebo).	II	Diarrhea reported in 2 patients receiving naloxone doses of 20% of daily morphine dose.
	Phase II: Open, dose-ranging	10	Cancer patients receiving regular oral opioids for pain control. Allowed to take other laxatives besides lactulose. Total daily dose of naloxone or placebo divided and given every 4 hours. Small bowel transit time measured with lactulose/hydrogen test.	Naloxone dose of ≥20% had a laxative effect. Two generalized withdrawal reactions occurred.	V	Patients received lactulose 15 mL orally for testing small bowel transit time; may have affected study results.

Key to Level of Evidence classification:
Level I   Randomized trials with low false-positive (alpha) and low false-negative (beta errors); high power
Level II   Randomized trials with high false-positive (alpha) and/or high false-negative (beta errors); low power
Level III   Nonrandomized concurrent cohort comparisons between contemporaneous patients who did and did not receive a given intervention
Level IV Nonrandomized historical cohort comparisons between current patients who did receive the intervention and patients (from the same institution or from the literature) who did not
Level V   Case series without control subjects

this patient population, anecdotal reports provide general guidelines for laxative therapy. While any of the pharmacologic measures listed in Table 2 may be helpful, the patient should be given choices and allowed to participate in the care whenever possible.[8] The role of each agent is described below

PREVENTION OF CONSTIPATION

Pharmacologic agents used primarily for the prevention of constipation include bulk-forming laxatives and stool softening agents in patients with normal peristaltic function. If peristalsis is severely impaired by disease, opioids, or anticholinergic agents, bulk forming laxatives may cause intestinal colic due to distention that does not result in defecation. Because abdominal distention and sensation of fullness may worsen preexisting anorexia, palliative care patients may not tolerate bulk-forming agents such as psyllium and methylcellulose. Risk of intestinal obstruction or impaction may increase in patients unable to consume the large quantities of fluid required with bulk-forming laxatives.[1] Stool softeners, such as docusate, may be effective for prevention of constipation in patients not taking drugs which impede peristalsis.

Patients initiating opioid therapy should be started on a laxative since constipation is a well-known effect of opioids.[1,4] Stimulant laxatives, e.g., standardized senna concentrate, bisacodyl, are the most appropriate laxatives for opioid-induced constipation. Some patients may experience abdominal colic with these drugs.[1] Patients with hard, dry stools while taking a stimulant laxative may require a combination of a stimulant and a stool softener for their preventative bowel regimen.[3] Prophylaxis with a liquid osmotic laxative, i.e., sorbitol or lactulose, may be helpful.[1] While the osmotic agents are equally efficacious, sorbitol may be better tolerated and is much less costly than lactulose.[4,9] In most cases, simply increasing the dose of stimulant is adequate and the osmotic agents are not needed

TREATMENT OF CONSTIPATION

Selection of the appropriate pharmacologic agent is guided by information obtained during the initial evaluation of the constipated

TABLE 2. Drug Therapy for Managing Constipation in Palliative Care[10,14-17]

Drug	Pharmacologic Effect	Dosing Regimen	AWP per Day of Therapy#
bisacodyl 5 mg tablet (Dulcolax) 10 mg rectal suppository	Stimulant laxative	T: 5-15 mg PO HS or T: 10 mg PR QD to BID prn	$0.03-0.09 $0.20-0.40
docusate sodium 100 mg capsule (Colace)	Stool softening surfactant	P: 1-2 capsules PO QD to BID	$0.03-0.09
docusate sodium 100 mg with casanthranol 30 mg per capsule (Peri-Colace, Doxidan)	Stool softening surfactant/stimulant combination	P: 1 capsule PO TID* T: 1-2 capsules up to BID (Liquid available: docusate sodium 60 mg, casanthranol 130 mg/15 mL)	$0.12 $0.08-0.16 $1.08-$2.19
docusate sodium 283 mg in glycerin base minienema (Therevac-SB)	Stool softening surfactant/osmotic laxative combination	T: 1 mini enema PR prn	$1.54
docusate sodium 50 mg with senna 187 mg tablet (Senokot-S)	Stool softening surfactant/stimulant combination	P: 1 tablet PO TID* T: 2 tablets QD-TID	$1.05 $0.70-2.10
glycerin rectal suppositories	Osmotic laxative	T: 1 suppository PR QD to BID prn	$0.08-0.16
lactulose	Osmotic laxative	T: 30 mL PO QD to BID	$1.98-3.97
milk of magnesia	Saline laxative	T: 30-60 mL PO QD to BID	$0.28-1.12
senna 187 mg tablet (Senokot)	Stimulant laxative	T: 2-4 tablets PO HS	$0.06-0.12
sodium phosphate/sodium biphosphate enema (Fleets Enema)	Saline laxative	T: 1 enema PR prn	$0.94
sorbitol	Osmotic laxative	P: 15-30 mL PO 1-4 times daily	$0.15-1.20

Abbreviations: BID = twice daily; HS = bedtime; P = regimen for prevention of constipation; PO = orally; PR = rectally; prn = as needed; QD = once daily; T = regimen for treatment of constipation; TID = three times daily
Average Wholesale Price, 1999 (cost to pharmacy)
* For patients receiving opioid analgesics

patient. Once constipation is relieved, the regimen should be modified as needed to prevent future episodes. If the rectum is full of hard feces, glycerin suppositories promote defecation by softening and lubricating the mass as well as stimulating defecation. A stool softener should be added to the patient's preventative regimen or the current dosage increased.

Patients with a full rectum containing soft feces may be treated with an oral stimulant laxative, e.g., standardized senna concentrate, bisacodyl, to stimulate bowel motility. If the rectum contains feces, bisacodyl suppositories may be ineffective since distribution of the active drug to the bowel mucosa may be decreased. A stimulant laxative should be added to the preventative regimen. If the stool is too soft, normal defecation or manual removal may become difficult.

If the rectum is empty, higher impaction and colonic loading may be present. Stimulants alone can be dangerous when there is obstruction or impaction. After softening the mass with an oil retention or aqueous enema, 1 to 2 bisacodyl suppositories given rectally will promote bowel peristalsis and defecation if the feces are soft. Addition of a glycerin suppository may be helpful in some cases. If the feces are hard, an oil retention enema may be required to soften the mass before defecation can occur.[3]

Enemas or manual evacuation may be necessary in patients unresponsive to oral laxatives or rectal suppositories.[1] Sodium phosphate/sodium biphosphate enemas and docusate sodium/glycerin mini-enemas are equal in efficacy although the latter may be preferred due to lack of phosphate content and decreased enema volume (< 5 mL vs. 130 mL).[10] Patients requiring disimpaction may benefit from pain medications or sedatives prior to the removal procedure.[3]

Lactulose has been evaluated for the treatment of constipation in terminally ill patients in two uncontrolled case series. Crowther (1978) reported that terminally ill patients receiving an average of 20 mL lactulose orally twice daily had a bowel movement every 2-3 days.[11] Patients described 71.5% of stools as easy to move, 20.7% as hard or difficult to pass, and 7.8% as loose. Over 40% of the loose stools occurred following administration of an enema or suppositories. Although the investigators stated that patients were frequently receiving opioid therapy, the percentage of patients on opioids was not reported. In a case series reported by Harris and Jackson,[12] lactulose therapy produced a bowel movement within 2 days in all of 8 patients. Six of the patients had experienced vincristine-induced constipation for 7 or more days. The other two patients received lactulose prophylactically following vincristine administration. No serum electrolyte changes were observed in any patient. The report did not specify whether patients were receiving opioids.

Lederle et al. compared the efficacy of sorbitol and lactulose in a double-blind, randomized crossover trial of 30 elderly men with chronic constipation not due to opioid analgesics.[9] The drugs were equally efficacious in relieving constipation, although nausea occurred significantly more frequently with lactulose than sorbitol ($p < 0.05$). A sequence effect was noted for one variable, number of days per week with bowel movements, possibly reflecting a difference between groups at randomization. Patient preference was evenly divided between sorbitol and lactulose. Based on lower cost and comparable efficacy, sorbitol may have a therapeutic advantage over lactulose. Although this study excluded patients receiving opioids, it suggests that sorbitol may be an alternative to lactulose in some patients.

Agra et al. compared the efficacy of senna and lactulose in 91 terminally ill cancer patients treated with opioids over a 27 day period.[13] They found no difference in defecation-free intervals or days without defecation. The authors concluded that senna is preferable due to similar side effects and markedly lower cost for senna.

Sykes evaluated oral naloxone in cancer patients with constipation due to regularly-scheduled oral morphine or diamorphine (heroin).[14] An apparent laxative effect was seen with a daily naloxone dose of ?20% of the daily morphine dose, divided and given every 4 hours. Withdrawal reactions were noted in some patients, as well as worsening of pain control.

Conclusion

Constipation is very common in palliative care patients. It occurs in approximately half of all patients with advanced cancer and in over 85% of patients receiving opioids. It may be a more frequent cause of severe distress than pain. Both non-pharmacologic and pharmacologic methods may be useful for the prevention and treatment of constipation. Thorough patient history and evaluation are key to selecting appropriate therapy. The goal of pharmacologic therapy is to prevent constipation and, failing that, to treat it. Because constipation occurs frequently with opioid analgesics, patients initiating opioid therapy should receive a laxative as a preventive measure. Senna appears to be the stimulating laxative of choice for patients receiving opioids.

SOME OPEN RESEARCH QUESTIONS

1. How much of a problem are adverse effects with drugs used to prevent and treat constipation?
2. When is the addition of a second laxative indicated in the management of constipation?
3. Does tolerance develop with long-term therapy for constipation?

REFERENCES

1. Burke A. The management of constipation in end-stage disease. Aust Fam Physician. 1994;23:1248-1253.

2. White T. Dealing with constipation. Nurs Times. 1995;91:57-60.

3. Sykes NP. Current approaches to the management of constipation. Cancer Surv. 1994;21:137-146.

4. Storey P. Symptom control in advanced cancer. Semin Oncol. 1994; December; 21:748-753.

5. Donnelly S, Walsh D. The symptoms of advanced cancer. Semin Oncol. 1995; 22:67-72.

6. Holmes S. Use of a modified symptom distress scale in assessment of the cancer patient. Int J Nurs Stud. 1989;26:69-79.

7. Anderson DM. Dorland's Illustrated Medical Dictionary. 28th ed. Philadelphia, PA: W.B. Saunders Company; 1994.

8. Cameron JC. Constipation related to narcotic therapy. A protocol for nurses and patients. Cancer Nursing. 1992;15:372-377.

9. Lederle FA, Busch DL, Mattox KM, West MJ, Aske DM. Cost-effective treatment of constipation in the elderly; A randomized double-blind comparison of sorbitol and lactulose. Am J Med. 1990;89:597-601.

10. Sykes NP. Constipation and diarrhoea. In: Doyle D, Hanks GWC, MacDonald N, eds. Oxford Textbook of Palliative Medicine. New York, NY: Oxford University Press; 1993:299-310.

11. Crowther AGO. Management of constipation in terminally ill patients. J Int Med Res. 1978;6:348-350.

12. Harris AC, Jackson JM. Lactulose in vincristine-induced constipation. Med J Aust. 1977;2:573-574.

13. Agra Y, Sacristan A, Gonzalez M, Ferrari M, Portugues A, Calvo M. Efficacy of senna versus lactulose in terminal cancer patients treated with opioids. J Pain Symptom Manage. 1998;15:1-7.

14. Sykes NP. An investigation of the ability of oral naloxone to correct opioid-related constipation in patients with advanced cancer. Palliat Med. 1996;10:135-144.

Delirium in Palliative Care Patients

Kenneth C. Jackson II
Arthur G. Lipman

SUMMARY. Delirium is commonly misunderstood in patients with advanced disease. It can present as a hyperactive, hypoactive or fluctuating disorder. Antineoplastic agents and other drugs may cause delirium as can some drug interactions. Potential causes are described. Evaluation instruments that have been used for this symptom are described. Some open research questions are listed. A management algorithm, evidence tables, and drug therapy tables which include drug costs are presented. *[Article copies available for a fee from The Haworth Document Delivery Service: 1-800-342-9678. E-mail address: getinfo@haworthpressinc. com <Website: http://www.haworthpressinc.com>]*

KEYWORDS. Delirium, agitation, restlessness, palliative care, terminal care, dying, opioids, prevention, supportive care, drug therapy, nonpharmacological therapy, etiology, evidence, costs, algorithm, systematic review, corticosteroids, anticholinergic agents, systematic review

---

Kenneth C. Jackson II, PharmD, is Manager of Clinical Pharmacy Services, St. Dominic-Jackson Memorial Hospital; and Clinical Assistant Professor, University of Mississippi School of Pharmacy, Jackson, MS.

Arthur G. Lipman, PharmD, is Professor, College of Pharmacy; Director of Clinical Pharmacology, Pain Management Center, University Hospitals and Clinics; Pain Medicine and Palliative Care Advisory Group, Huntsman Cancer Center; University of Utah Health Sciences Center, Salt Lake City, UT.

Address correspondence to: Arthur G. Lipman, PharmD, College of Pharmacy and Pain Management Center, 30 S 2000 E RM 258, University of Utah Health Sciences Center, Salt Lake City, UT 84112-5820 (E-mail: alipman@pharm.utah.edu).

[Haworth co-indexing entry note]: "Delirium in Palliative Care Patients." Jackson, Kenneth C. II, and Arthur G. Lipman. Co-published simultaneously in *Journal of Pharmaceutical Care in Pain & Symptom Control* (Pharmaceutical Products Press, an imprint of The Haworth Press, Inc.) Vol. 7, No. 4, 1999, pp. 59-70; and: *Evidence Based Symptom Control in Palliative Care: Systematic Reviews and Validated Clinical Practice Guidelines for 15 Common Problems in Patients with Life Limiting Disease* (ed: Arthur G. Lipman, Kenneth C. Jackson II, and Linda S. Tyler) Pharmaceutical Products Press, an imprint of The Haworth Press, Inc., 2000, pp. 59-70. Single or multiple copies of this article are available for a fee from The Haworth Document Delivery Service [1-800-342-9678, 9:00 a.m. - 5:00 p.m. (EST). E-mail address: getinfo@haworthpressinc.com].

Algorithm for Managing Delirium

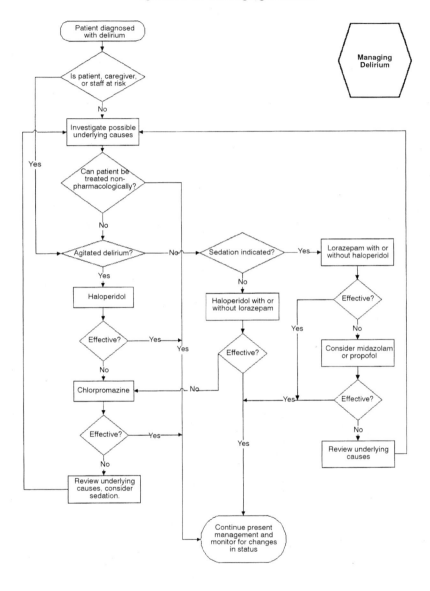

Challenges from delirium in palliative care encompass direct patient care and care of the patient's family and other caregivers. This care can have a profound impact on the quality of life for all involved. The goal of therapy is to enhance the mental, physical, and spiritual well being of not only the patient, but all involved in the patient's care.

Confusion about the management of delirium arises from misunderstanding of the definition for the disease state. The DSM-IV criteria for diagnosing delirium help to understand this disease. Delirium is a disturbance resulting from an altered mental state described in terms of disrupted consciousness and impaired cognition.

Delirium is described using varied terminology in the literature. Terms such as agitation, confusional states, encephalopathy, organic mental disorders, and terminal restlessness are found throughout the palliative care literature. When referring to terminal restlessness, a quantitative time frame should be defined. Treatment approaches will depend on the subtleties of defining the patient's delirium, especially as it relates to agitation.

Delirium differs from dementia which is chronic and progressive cognitive impairment. Delirium is more acute, can be reversed, has a fluctuating course, and is primarily a disorder of level of consciousness. These two disorders are not mutually exclusive. Patients with dementia may be predisposed to delirium, and as such difficulties may arise in diagnosis and management.

POSSIBLE ETIOLOGIES[1-3]

Delirium can arise from multiple causes including:

- environmental factors
- metabolic encephalopathy
- electrolyte abnormalities
- infection/sepsis
- hematological abnormalities
- nutritional deficits
- paraneoplastic syndromes
- primary brain malignancy and metastases to the central nervous system
- seizures
- hypoxia
- medications

Attention to the underlying source should provide the best treatment approach for most patients. However, when the underlying cause is not readily reversible, management may require pharmacological intervention.

Many drugs are well known to elicit delirium in the terminal patient. Opioids, anticholinergic agents, corticosteroids, and antineoplastic agents are known to contribute to the delirious state.[1-6] Numerous other drugs and drug combinations can contribute to the confusion seen in these patients. Theses include the following.

Antineoplastic Agents Associated with Causing Delirium[1-4,7]

altretamine	bleomycin	carmustine
cis-platinum	cytosine arabinoside	dexamethasone
fludarabine	5-FU (fluorouracil)	hydroxyurea
ifosfamide	interferon	interleukine-2
l-asparaginase	methotrexate	prednisone
procarbazine	Vinblastine	vincristine

Examples of Other Medications Associated with Delirium[1-8]

acyclovir	amantadine	antihistamines
atropine	bromocriptine	bupropion
beta-lactam antibiotics	carbamazepine	chloral hydrate
cimetidine	dexamethasone	digoxin
ganciclovir	indomethacin	lidocaine
methyldopa	mexilitine	penicillin
prednisone	quinidone	quinolones
ranitidine	saquinavir	selegine
tocainide	topiramate	valproic acid

Examples of Drug-Drug Interactions Implicated in Delirium[2,3,6-8]

disulfiram/metronidazole:	reports of confusion and pychotic behavior
haloperidol/carbamazepine:	increased metabolism of haloperidol
haloperidol/methyldopa:	may cause confusion/disorientation
haloperidol/lithium:	enhanced lithium toxicity
ace inhibitors/lithium:	decreased lithium excretion (toxicity)
diuretics/lithium:	decreased lithium excretion (toxicity) with chronic use
methyldopa/lithium:	lithium toxicity
NSAIDs/lithium:	decreased lithium excretion (toxicity)
	(may be less likely with ibuprofen, nabumetone, or sulindac)
phenytoin/lithium:	lithium toxicity without necessarily elevated serum levels
MAO inhibitors/SSRI's:	serotonin syndrome

NON-PHARMACOLOGICAL APPROACH

Placing patients in a quiet, safe, and supportive environment is the first step in managing delirium. This assists in reorienting the patient. Attempts should be made to treat any underlying causes for the delirium prior to initiating drug therapy. Correction of nutritional deficits or electrolyte abnormalities is relatively easy, and often obviates the need for drug therapy. However, certain metabolic abnormalities, e.g., liver failure, may not be reversible. With brain tumors or metastases, reduction of intracranial pressure may help to resolve delirium. Steroids used to decrease intracranial pressure may precipitate a delirious state. The possibility of drug-drug interactions being causative should be investigated. A thorough review of the patient's medication profile and laboratory indices may potential insight into causes.

PHARMACOTHERAPY

Using medications in the treatment of delirium is generally necessary prior to, or following, examination of potential underlying etiologies. Haloperidol is often cited as the drug of choice for delirium.[1-4,9-11] The vast majority of literature in this area is anecdotal. There are numerous review articles available.[1,12-18]

Prior to selecting a drug to use in the patient with delirium, it is useful to ascertain what components of the disease process are currently being manifested. Patients may or may not exhibit signs of agitation, i.e., have hyperactive or hypoactive delirium.[3,6] This will effect the approach to therapy. In this regard, many patients with delirium may present in a confused state and benzodiazepines may only exacerbate the condition. Many patients with hypoactive delirium probably go undiagnosed.[3] Another relevant component relates to the patient's life expectancy. The approach to managing delirium is greatly influenced by the perceived urgency for an intervention, as well as the anticipated life expectancy. Patients in their last days of life may be appropriate candidates for more intensive treatment of their delirium.[17,19-23] The opposite may be true if the symptoms are not distressing to the patient or family.

Haloperidol

The American College of Critical Care Medicine has stated that haloperidol should be considered the preferred agent for treating critically ill adults with delirium.[10] Breitbart and colleagues reported in a prospective, randomized, double blind trial that both haloperidol and chlorpromazine improved delirium symptoms in hospitalized AIDS patients, as measured by the Delirium Rating Scale.[24] A third arm using lorazepam as a single entity was stopped due to adverse effects, including increased confusion. A series of case reports has been published in which patients with agitated delirium responded favorably to treatment with haloperidol.[17] In a retrospective analysis of 39 patients with advanced cancer, haloperidol adequately controlled the delirium in 8 (21%) cases.[9] Adding lorazepam to haloperidol provided control in an additional 10 (26%) of patients.

Chlorpromazine

McIver and colleagues reported a prospective analysis of chlorpromazine in patients with terminal restlessness.[25] In their analysis, 18 of 20 patients had complete symptom relief prior to death. The other two patients were noted to have had partial relief at death. Patients received chlorpromazine via the rectal or intravenous route. In the previously mentioned trial by Breitbart and colleagues, chlorpromazine (oral or intramuscular) was shown to improve symptoms of delirium.[24]

Midazolam

Midazolam was used in 10 of 39 patients to control delirium by sedation.[9] In 9 of these patients, symptom control was achieved with subcutaneous midazolam. In a retrospective analysis of 86 patients who required subcutaneous midazolam, 85 patients achieved symptom relief.[22] Fainsinger and Bruera reported a case in which a patient was refractory to other treatments.[21] The clinicians were able to provide symptom relief with subcutaneous midazolam, at the expense of marked sedation. This may be beneficial in some patients with terminal agitation. Midazolam administration requires close monitoring, and as such may not be an appropriate choice for the majority of palliative patients.

Propofol

There are several case reports of propofol being used in the management of terminal delirium.[19-21] Propofol was initially developed as an intravenous anesthetic induction agent. Both midazolam and propofol have been suggested as preferred agents for short-term treatment of anxiety in critically ill adults.[10] Propofol has a pharmacokinetic advantage over midazolam in that the level of sedation can be more readily controlled or reversed. Propofol is a lipid based emulsion and as such provides a growth medium for microorganisms. The lipid emulsion does provide a caloric load (1.1 kcal/mL) which could be a factor in long-term use of this medication. Additionally, if propofol were to be used for an extended period of time, the patient's liver function tests would require monitoring. Propofol must be given intravenously and many clinicians may be wary of its use in the home. As with midazolam, propofol appears to have a very limited indication in palliative care.

CONCLUSION

The evidence for using neuroleptics in the palliative care population is scarce. Selection of chlorpromazine versus haloperidol is primarily based on anecdote. The one controlled clinical trial has shown these medications to be equally efficacious.[24] Factors to be considered in selecting therapy include the subtype of delirium, route of administration, and side effect profile. The severity of symptoms and the patient's life expectancy will influence therapy. Studies of atypical antipsychotics medications, e.g., olanzapine, risperidone, might provide further insight into the management of delirium in palliative care.

Clinicians should remain alert for manifestations of delirium in patients near the end of life. To date, no tool for detecting delirium has been developed in palliative care patients. Numerous tools, e.g., The Memorial Delirium Assessment Scale, Delirium Rating Scale[26,27] have been validated in other patient populations. Smith and colleagues have written a very useful review of instruments used for detecting, diagnosing, and rating delirium.[28] Development of a tool specifically for the palliative care population may assist practitioners in detecting and differentiating delirium in the future.

TABLE 1. Drug Therapy for Managing Delirium in Palliative Care Evidence Tables

Reference	Study Design	n	Intervention	Results	Level of Evidence	Comments
Chlorpromazine (Thorazine)						
Breitbart see haloperidol	Prospective Double-blind Randomized	30	Haloperidol (n = 11) vs. chlorpromazine (n = 13) vs. lorazepam (n = 6). Mean chlorpromazine dose of 50 mg the first 24 hours. Mean 24-hour maintenance dose was 36 mg.	Chlorpromazine and haloperidol improved symptoms over the first 24 hours, as measured by the Delirium Rating Scale. No significant changes noted after 48 hours.	II	Lorazepam arm stopped early due to adverse effects.
McIver (1994)	Descriptive	20	Chlorpromazine was dosed Q4H in 18 patients, Q6H in one patient, and Q12H in one patient (Median starting doses 25 mg PR, 12.5 mg IV). Patients had dyspnea, pain, and terminal restlessness. Patients were equally distributed between home (PR) and hospital (IV).	Patients received a median of 2 doses prior to death. Eighteen patients had complete symptom relief and 2 had partial relief prior to death.	V	Patients had rapid relief with small doses, especially in the elderly.
Midazolam (Versed)						
Fainsinger (1992)	Descriptive Case Report	1	Patient refractory to haloperidol, haloperidol plus lorazepam, and methotrimeprazine (no longer available in the U.S.).	Delirium was controlled with midazolam 1-4 mg/hr by continuous SC infusion.	V	Patient experience marked sedation with regimen.
Burke (1991)	Descriptive Retrospective	86	Midazolam 2.5-10 mg SC bolus Q2H or via SC infusion (20-60 mg/d).	Stated to be effective in 85 of the 86 patients	V	Patient failure noted after removal of SC access.
Propofol (Diprivan)						
Mercadante (1995)	Descriptive Case Report	1	Patient received a 20 mg loading dose followed by 50-70 mg/hr.	Delirium was well controlled prior to death. Patient died 8 hours after the infusion began.	V	Patient died peacefully

Moyle (1995)	Descriptive Case Report	2	Patient 1: Initiated at 10 mg/hr and escalated to 200 mg/hr over 9 days. Patient 2: Infusion begun at 100 mg/hr, and ranged from 100 mg/hr to 400 mg/hr over next 4 days.	Patient 1: Required dose escalations secondary to tachyphylaxis. Patient died peacefully on day 9. Patient 2: Had fluctuating level of consciousness while on midazolam. Tolerated propofol without problems and died peacefully on day 4.	V	Author proposed protocol for propofol use.

Haloperidol (Haldol)

Breitbart (1996)	Prospective Double-blind Randomized	30	Haloperidol (n = 11) vs. chlorpromazine (n = 13) vs. lorazepam (n = 6). Mean haloperidol dose first 24 hours was 2.8 mg. Mean maintenance dose 1.4 mg/day	Haloperidol and chlorpromazine treatment arms showed improvement in symptoms over first 24 hours, as measured by the Delirium Rating Scale. No significant changes noted after 48 hours	II	Lorazepam arm stopped early due to adverse effects.
De Stoutz (1995)	Descriptive Case reports	4	Report of 4 patients who received haloperidol, in addition to numerous other changes in their treatment regimen.	All four patients had a satisfactory resolution of their delirium.	V	All 4 patients had potentially reversible causes.
Stiefel (1992)	Descriptive Retrospective analysis	39	Retrospective analysis of 39 patients who presented with delirium. Delirium was controlled in 23 patients	Haloperidol (PO or SC) effective in 8/23 patients, and 10/23 patients when combined with lorazepam.	V	Report did not state haloperidol dose required.

Key to Level of Evidence Classification:
Level I   Randomized trials with low false-positive (alpha) and low false-negative (beta errors); high power
Level II   Randomized trials with high false-positive (alpha) and/or high false-negative (beta errors); low power
Level III Nonrandomized concurrent cohort comparisons between contemporaneous patients who did and did not receive a given intervention
Level IV Nonrandomized historical cohort comparisons between current patients who did receive the intervention and patients (from the same institution or from the literature) who did not
Level V   Case series without control subjects

TABLE 2. Pharmacotherapeutic Options in Treating Delirium[1-4,7,8,10,14,19,20,22,24,25]

Presentation	Drug/Regimen of Choice	Alternative Medications	AWP per Day of Therapy#	Other
Hyperactive delirium	haloperidol (IM, IV, PO) Initial: 0.5-1.0 mg PO and repeat dose as titrated against response. Range: 2-100 mg/day or chlorpromazine (IM, IV, PO, PR) Initial: 30 mg PO and repeat in 1-4 hours as indicated by response. Range: 30-800 mg/day	thioridazine (PO) Initial: 50-100 mg PO TID Range: 50-800 mg/day or haloperidol (IM, IV, PO) plus lorazepam Initial: 0.44 mg/kg IV/IM Q2-4H PRN Range: 2-10 mg/day	haloperidol: 1 mg PO qid $0.08/day 5 mg IM/IV qid $11.85/day chlorpromazine: 25 mg PO tid $0.18/day 25 mg PR tid $8.87/day 25 mg IV tid $21.77 lorazepam: 2 mg IV/IM Q6H $21.53	Consider side effects when selecting primary agent (neurologic vs. cardiovascular effects) Parenteral dose usually 50% of oral dose Geriatric patients use initial dose of 20-25% (haloperidol, chlorpromazine, thioridazine) Haloperidol better tolerated in doses less than 20 mg/day
Hypoactive delirium	haloperidol (IM, IV, PO)	thioridazine (PO) or chlorpromazine (IM, IV, PO, PR)	thioridazine: 50 mg PO tid $0.16/day	Avoid agents with sedative properties (may add to confusion), especially benzodiazepines
Fluctuating delirium (hypo/hyperactive)	haloperidol (IM, IV, PO)	chlorpromazine (IM, IV, PO, PR) or thioridazine (PO)		Could use chlorpromazine in lieu of haloperidol if sedative properties warranted
Delirium requiring sedation	midazolam (IV,SC) Initial: 0.03 mg/kg bolus Range: 2-10 mg/day SC	propofol (IV) Initial: 10 mg/hr Range: 5-70 mg/hr	midazolam: 10 mg IV/SQ per day $19.07/day propofol: 5 mg IV per hour $7.71/day 70 mg IV per hour $107.92/day	Agents only indicated when sedation required, i.e., terminal restlessness or refractory to other measures. Propofol is a lipid-based emulsion, exercise care to prevent contamination. Titrate dose to response Monitor respiratory and neurological status closely

Average Wholesale Price, 1999 (cost to pharmacy)

SOME OPEN RESEARCH QUESTIONS

1. How common is hypoactive delirium in palliative care patients?
2. When is the addition of lorazepam to haloperidol generally indicated for management of delirium in palliative care patients?
3. Is subcutaneous midazolam cost effective for this indication?
4. What is the role of propofol in managing terminal delirium?
5. What is the role of the atypical neuroleptics for this indication?

REFERENCES

1. Roth AJ, Breitbart W. Psychiatric emergencies in terminally ill cancer patients. Pain and Palliat Care. 1996;10:235-259.

2. Hanks GW, Portenoy RK, MacDonald N, O'Neill WM. Difficult pain problems. In: Doyle D, Hanks GWC, MacDonald N, eds. Oxford Textbook of Pallitive Medicine. New York: Oxford University Press; 1993:257-274.

3. Ingham JM, Caraceni AT. Delirium. In: Berger AM, Portenoy RK, Weissman DE, eds. Principles and Practice of Supportive Oncology. Philadelphia, PA: Lippincott-Raven; 1998:477-496.

4. Massie MJ, Holland JC. The cancer patient with pain: psychiatric complications and their management. Med Clin North Am. 1987;71:243-258.

5. Martin EW. Confusion in the terminally ill:recognition and management. Am J Hsop Pall Care. 1990;7:20-24.

6. Trzepacz PT. The neuropathogenesis of delirium: a need to focus our research. Psychosomatics. 1994;35:374-391.

7. Lacy C, Armstrong LL, Ingrim N, Lance LL. Drug Information Handbook. 3rd ed: Lexi-comp; 1995.

8. Crismon ML, Dorson PG. Delirium. In Pharmacotherapy 3rd edition, Dipiro J. Talbert R, Yee G, et al., eds, Stamford CT. Appleton and Lange, 1997.

9. Stiefel F, Fainsinger R, Bruera E. Acute confusional states in patients with advanced cancer. J Pain Symptom Manage. 1992;7:94-98.

10. Shapiro BA, Warren J, Egol AB, et al. Practice parameters for intravenous analgesia and sedation for adult patients in the intensive care unit: an executive summary. Crit Care Med. 1995;23:1596-1600.

11. Gelfand SB, Indelicato J, Benjamin J. Using intravenous haloperidol to control delirium. Hosp and Comm Psychiatry. 1992;43:215.

12. Fainsinger RL, Tapper M, Bruera E. A perspective on the management of delirium in terminally ill patients on a palliative care unit. J Palliat Care. 1993;9:4-8.

13. Breitbart W, Jacobsen PB. Psychiatric symptom management in terminal care. Clin Geriatr Med. 1996;12:329-347.

14. Bluestine S, Lesko L. Psychotropic medications in oncology and in AIDS patients. Adv Psychosom Med. 1994;21:107-137.

15. Adams F. Neuropsychiatric evaluation and treatment of delirium in the critically ill cancer patient. The Cancer Bulletin. 1984;36:156-160.

16. Caraceni A. Delirium in palliative care. Eur J Palliat Care. 1995;2:62-67.

17. de Stoutz ND, Tapper M, Fainsinger RL. Reversible delirium in terminally ill patients. J Pain Symptom Manage. 1995;10:249-253.

18. Stiefel F, Razavi D. Common psychiatric disorders in cancer patients II. Anxiety and acute confusional states. Support Care Cancer. 1994;2:233-237.

19. Mercadante S, De Conno F, Ripamonti C. Propofol in terminal care. J Pain Symptom Manage. 1995;10:639-642.

20. Moyle J. The use of propofol in palliative medicine. J Pain Symptom Manage. 1995;10:643-646.

21. Fainsinger R, Bruera E. Treatment of delirium in a terminally ill patient. J Pain Symptom Manage. 1992;7:54-56.

22. Burke AL, Diamond PL, Hulbert J, Yeatman J, Farr EA. Terminal restlessness–its management and the role of midazolam. Med J Aust. 1991;155:485-487.

23. Burke AL. Palliative care: an update on "terminal restlessness." Med J Aust. 1997;166:39-42.

24. Breitbart W, Marotta R, Platt M, et al. A double-blind trial of haloperidol, chlorpromazine, and lorazepam in the treatment of delirium in hospitalized AIDS patients. Am J Psychiatry. 1996;153:231-237.

25. McIver B, Walsh D, Nelson K. The use of chlorpromazine for symptom control in dying cancer patients. J Pain Sympt Manage. 1994;9:341-345.

26. Trzepacz PT, Baker RW, Greenhouse J. A Symptom Rating Scale for delirium. Psychiatry Research. 1988;23:89-97.

27. Breitbart W, Rosenfeld B, Roth A, Smith MJ, Cohen K, Passik S. The Memorial Delirium Assessment Scale. J Pain Symptom Manage. 1997;12:128-137.

28. Smith MJ, Breitbart WS, Platt MM. A critique of instruments and methods used to detect, diagnose, and rate delirium. J Pain Symptom Manage. 1995;10:35-77.

Depression in Palliative Care Patients

Andrew C. Martin
Kenneth C. Jackson II

SUMMARY. Depression is common in patients with advanced, irreversible disease, but it is not normal. Many drugs and morbid states have been associated with depression. Psychotherapy, cognitive therapy, and electroconvulsive therapy, as well as pharmacotherapy may be helpful. The use of antidepressants and psychostimulants to manage depression in terminally ill patients is reviewed. Evaluation instruments that have been used to assess depression in this population are described. Some open research questions are listed. A treatment algorithm, evidence tables, and drug therapy tables which include drug costs are presented. *[Article copies available for a fee from The Haworth Document Delivery Service: 1-800-342-9678. E-mail address: getinfo@ haworthpressinc.com <Website: http://www.haworthpressinc.com>]*

KEYWORDS. Depression, agitation, insomnia, affect, mood, energy, apathy, anger, withdrawal, noncompliance, palliative care, terminal care, dying, supportive care, non-pharmacological therapy, drug therapy, etiology, evidence, costs, algorithm, inhibitors, psychotherapy, education, electroconvulsive therapy (ECT), psychostimulants, dextroamphetamine, methylphenidate, pemoline, tricyclic antidepressants (TCA), amitriptyline, desipramine, norptriptyline, doxepin, diazepam, bupropion, selective serotonin reuptake inhibitors, SSRI, fluoxetine, fluvoxamine, paroxetine, sertraline, citalopram, mirtazapine, venlafaxine, thrioridazine, trazodone, nefazodone, amoxapine, monoamine oxidase inhibitors (MAOI), phenelzine, tranylcypromine

Andrew C. Martin, PharmD, is Assistant Professor, School of Pharmacy, Ferris State College, Big Rapids, MI.

Kenneth C. Jackson II, PharmD, is Manager of Clinical Pharmacy Services, St. Dominic-Jackson Memorial Hospital; and Clinical Assistant Professor, University of Mississippi School of Pharmacy, Jackson, MS.

Address correspondence to: Arthur G. Lipman, PharmD, College of Pharmacy and Pain Management Center, 30 S 2000 E RM 258, University of Utah Health Sciences Center, Salt Lake City, UT 84112-5820 (E-mail: alipman@pharm.utah.edu).

[Haworth co-indexing entry note]: "Depression in Palliative Care Patients." Martin, Andrew C., and Kenneth C. Jackson II. Co-published simultaneously in *Journal of Pharmaceutical Care in Pain & Symptom Control* (Pharmaceutical Products Press, an imprint of The Haworth Press, Inc.) Vol. 7, No. 4, 1999, pp. 71-89; and: *Evidence Based Symptom Control in Palliative Care: Systematic Reviews and Validated Clinical Practice Guidelines for 15 Common Problems in Patients with Life Limiting Disease* (ed: Arthur G. Lipman, Kenneth C. Jackson II, and Linda S. Tyler) Pharmaceutical Products Press, an imprint of The Haworth Press, Inc., 2000, pp. 71-89. Single or multiple copies of this article are available for a fee from The Haworth Document Delivery Service [1-800-342-9678, 9:00 a.m. - 5:00 p.m. (EST). E-mail address: getinfo@haworthpressinc.com].

Algorithm for Managing Depression

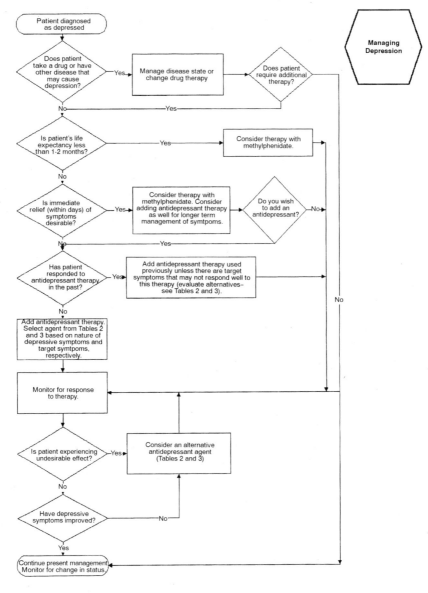

Depression in terminally ill patients is commonly thought to be a normal and appropriate adaptation to the prognosis or to result from the underlying pathology. While emotional distress is a natural response to being confronted with the finality of death; depression is a maladaptive and possibly harmful reaction. The acceptance of depression as normal has slowed the critical evaluation of the management of depression in palliative care patients. The somatic symptoms of depression are difficult to separate from the effects of the disease state.[1,2] Individual personality, existing support network, and medical problems impact the degree of psychological stress any given patient will experience.[3]

Evidence regarding the treatment of depression in palliative care patients primarily consists of case reports and studies involving medications unavailable in the United States. The rationale for choosing therapy is usually based on extrapolations made from the general psychiatric and medical literature and from assumptions of a pharmacologic class effect. The following discussion is a summary of the methods used to identify and manage depression in palliative care patients. Table 1 presents the published evidence.

INCIDENCE

Data on terminally ill patients are limited, but several studies have evaluated the incidence of depression specifically in terminally ill cancer patients. Minagawa et al. evaluated 93 Japanese patients with terminal cancer to determine the prevalence of psychiatric disorders. Psychiatric morbidity was diagnosed in 53.7% of patients; major depression accounted for 3.2% of this group.[4] Another study found an incidence of 13% to 26% for major or minor depression in terminally ill cancer patients depending on the diagnostic screening tools used in the assessment.[5]

IDENTIFICATION

Palliative care patients typically present with multiple symptoms. Weakness, fatigue, and loss of vitality are well known sequelae of cancer treatment. These symptoms may continue when patients are not

TABLE 1. Therapy in the Management of Depression in Palliative Care Patients–Evidence Table

Reference	Study Design	n	Intervention	Results	Level of Evidence	Comments
Cohen (1994)[26]	Descriptive Case Reports	3	Three patients sat approximately 45 cm from a 5000 lux wide-spectrum white light for 0.5-3 hours each morning for two weeks.	All patients rated mood and energy as moderately improved (2) or very much improved (1) as assessed by a nine point Global Assessment Scale	V	No patient had seasonal affective disorder or had a identifiable pharmacologic cause for depression
Johnston (1972)[27]	Prospective Double Blind, Randomized	50	Twenty-five patients received thioridazine 25 mg TID and 25 patients received matching placebo TID for six weeks.	The thioridazine arm achieved a significant decreases in symptom scores for anxiety-tension, depression, restlessness, and insomnia at one week, but after six weeks, depressive mood and restlessness symptom scores were not significantly different from placebo group.	II	Patients had diagnosis of mixed anxiety-depressive state. Three patients in the treatment arm died and were excluded from analysis. No adverse effects reported, but only 14 of 22 original thioridazine patients and 15 of original 25 placebo patients included in analysis at six weeks.
Maisami (1985)[28]	Descriptive, Case Reports	3	Amitriptyline and haloperidol were administered; doses and schedules were not delineated.	Within one week, satisfactory improvements occurred in mood (including depression, anxiety, agitation, anger, and social withdrawal), and narcotic and benzodiazepine use stopped.	V	Discontinuation of treatment occurred on two of the cases resulting in return to baseline.
Sheehan (1994)[29]	Descriptive, Case Report	1	Therapy was initiated with amitriptyline 50 mg QHS without benefit and changed to nortriptyline 25 mg QHS that was titrated to 45 mg QHS.	Patient left hospice care to pursue active curative treatment.	V	

Study	Type	N	Methods	Level	Results
Malitz (1972)[30]	Descriptive, Case Report	1	Nortriptyline 25-50 mg TID, diazepam 5 mg 3-5 doses daily, and flurazepam at HS were administered for depression, agitation, and insomnia. Schedules increased over patients course of therapy.	V	Patient started medications and psychotherapy before cancer diagnosis. Both therapies resumed after diagnosis of and surgery for advanced cancer. Therapy discontinued before diagnosis but resulted in eventual return of anxiety and depression. Medication and counseling managed the depression and anxiety until her death seven months later.
Macleod (1998)[31]	Descriptive, Case Series	26	Methylphenidate was initiated at 10 mg/day and titrated to 5-20 mg/day. Treatment was continued for a minimum of five days and discontinued six weeks after initiation or three weeks after response.	V	Mean dose and duration were 17.7 mg and 21 days, respectively. Seven patients (27%) achieved moderate or marked response by clinical global impression scale. Symptoms that responded include euthanasia request, suicidal ideation, fear of impending death, quality of time spent with relatives and anhedonia.
Breitbart (1992)[32]	Descriptive, Case Reports	4	Two of four patients were terminally ill. They received pemoline 18.75 mg QD initially, titrated over 4-7 days to 37.5 m BID	V	Terminally ill patients benefited from psychostimulant therapy by resolution of suicidal ideation, improved mood, and enjoyment of social interactions. Clinical global impression scales used to assess mood only. Marked improvement indicated complete or nearly complete remission achieved. Moderate improvement indicated that several symptoms improved without complete remission. One patient discontinued methylphenidate due to tachycardia; another experienced acute delirium thought to be due to a paraneoplastic phenomenon not therapy. Pemoline was indicated because one patient had a high risk of bowel obstruction and other fatigue and psychomotor retardation.

Key to Level of Evidence classification:

Level I   Randomized trials with low false-positive (alpha) and low false-negative (beta errors); high power
Level II   Randomized trials with high false-positive (alpha) and/or high false-negative (beta errors); low power
Level III   Nonrandomized concurrent cohort comparisons between contemporaneous patients who did and did not receive a given intervention
Level IV   Nonrandomized historical cohort comparisons between current patients who did receive the intervention and patients (from the same institution or from the literature) who did not
Level V   Case series without control subjects

75

undergoing active treatment, and they can markedly decrease quality of life.[6] Frank mood changes are the most easily identifiable signs of depression. When patients present with more subtle signs such as poor compliance, unwillingness to cooperate with health care professionals, social withdrawal, anger, or apathy, they should also be evaluated for depression.[1] Dysphoric mood, feelings of helplessness or hopelessness, loss of self-esteem, feelings of worthlessness or guilt, anhedonia, and suicidal ideation are key indicators of depression.[7]

Identifying factors that predispose patients to depression may improve the ability to prevent patient suffering. The presence of pain and other physical symptoms of disease tends to increase the likelihood that a patient will develop depression. This is especially true as the number and severity of physical symptoms increase. Cancer of the central nervous system is more likely to promote the development of psychiatric disorders than other types of cancer. Pancreatic cancer has been shown to be a more likely cause of depression than other abdominal cancers. A history of psychiatric problems or substance abuse may also predispose patients to depression.[3]

Many organic sources have been identified as possible causes of depression and should be addressed when possible before initiating therapy for depression. Drugs (opioids, psychotropics, corticosteroids, cytotoxic agents), infection, macroscopic brain pathology (primary or secondary tumor), Alzheimer's Disease, cerebrovascular disease, HIV dementia, metabolic disorders (dehydration, electrolyte disturbance, hypercalcemia, organ failure), and drug withdrawal may contribute to the onset of depression.[2,7-9]

Drugs Associated with Depression[7,10]		
acyclovir	amphetamine-like drugs	anabolic steroids
anticonvulsants	asparaginase	baclofen
barbiturates	benzodiazepines	beta-adrenergic blockers
bromocriptine	calcium-channel blockers	clonidine
corticosteroids	cycloserine	cyproterone
dapsone	digitalis glycosides	disopyramide
disulfiram	estrogens	fluoroquinolone antibiotics
H$_2$-receptor blockers	HMG-COA reductase inhibitors	interferon alfa
isotretinoin	levodopa	mefloquine
methyldopa	metoclopramide	metrizamide
metronidazole	NSAIDs	opioids
pergolide	phenylpropanolamine	procarbazine
progestins	sulfonamides	tamoxifen
thiazide diuretics	vinblastine	vincristine

In addition to difficulty in distinguishing somatic effects of drugs and diseases from depression, diagnosis of depression is hindered by the unreliability of available tools. Standard methods of evaluating patients for depression were developed with the physically well patient in mind. Chochinov et al. screened 197 terminally ill patients for the presence of depression using a single-item interview, a two-item interview, a Beck Depression Inventory (short form), or a visual analog scale. They determined that multiple-item tools were no more likely to diagnose depression than simply asking the patient if he or she is depressed. Furthermore, asking patients if they obtain pleasure in activities did not increase the sensitivity of the diagnosis over the one-item screen nor did it increase false negative results.[11] The authors recommend using the Beck Depression Inventory and a visual analog scale to assess change, to provide quantifiable information, and for diagnosis when patients cannot be interviewed. The Hospital Anxiety and Depression Scale excludes somatic symptoms of depression and may provide a greater degree of specificity for palliative care patients.[12]

NON-PHARMACOLOGIC MANAGEMENT

Psychotherapy is an important component of treatment. Most patients need to talk about their feelings, beliefs, and regrets as they relate to death and dying. It is the process of dying that most patients fear.[13] Due to the emergent nature of the situation, crisis intervention methods work well. Emotional and social support are important aspects of therapy. Simply providing a listening ear be therapeutic. Educational interventions and cognitive exercises such as problem-solving therapy, help patients to keep their thoughts rational, clear, and directed, and help them to maintain a feeling of control over the situation.[14]

Electroconvulsive therapy (ECT) is another effective, non-pharmacologic treatment option. It is safe and effective for use in medically ill patients, but no studies have evaluated its use in terminally ill patients.[7,15] ECT may be considered for patients with suicidal or psychotic features or contraindications to drug therapy.

PHARMACOLOGIC MANAGEMENT

Review articles presenting treatment guidelines for depression in palliative care patients are based on practice experience. Treatment is recommended when the patient presents with a definite depressive syndrome or depressive adjustment reaction lasting longer than a few weeks.[2,8,16-19] These reviews mainly discuss the role of tricyclic antidepressants and selective serotonin reuptake inhibitors. It is not clear to what extent bupropion, trazodone, nefazodone, venlafaxine, and the remaining miscellaneous antidepressants are useful in managing depression in palliative care patients. The lack of consensus is likely due to the paucity of evidence supporting the use of these agents.

Psychostimulants

The first patient factor that should be considered when choosing therapy is life expectancy. Patients who are expected to live for more than 2 months may have time to respond to antidepressive agents. If a patient's life expectancy is less than two months, a psychostimulant will relieve the patient's symptoms in a more timely manner than an antidepressant. Correspondingly, if more immediate relief is desired than an antidepressant *per se* can accomplish, a psychostimulant is an appropriate alternative.

Not only do psychostimulants provide a rapid onset of action, they may also stimulate appetite and promote a sense of well being. Their "energizing" effect may be especially desirable for patients experiencing debilitating weakness, fatigue, or drug therapy-associated CNS depression.. Patients who have psychomotor slowing, mild cognitive impairment, and/or dysphoric mood may also benefit from a psychostimulant.[7,19]

Despite the many positive effects of the psychostimulants, there are several adverse effects associated with their use. Nervousness, overstimulation, insomnia, euphoria, mood lability, mild increase in blood pressure and heart rate, tremor, dyskinesias, motor tics, paranoia, and exacerbation of an underlying confusional state may occur.[20]

Three psychostimulants are available in the United States, dextroamphetamine, methylphenidate and pemoline. Some clinicians find pemoline easier to use. This may be due to the fact that pemoline is less potent and easier to titrate to the desired effect. However, reports of hepatotoxicity resulted in the Food and Drug Administration initiating a "Dear Heath Professional letter" in 1999 advising that this drug should be used only when there is informed written consent assuring that the patient is aware of the potential liver toxicity. Pemoline is available in a chewable tablet formulation offering another alternative for patients who cannot swallow. Due to the hepatotoxicity, it does not have a place in palliative care.

Dextroamphetamine and methylphenidate can potentiate the analgesic effect of opioids and counter opioid induced sedation as well. As a result, these psychostimulants may permit patients to continue communicating with family and friends without compromising analgesic control. They may also be used to counter the sedating effect of antidepressive agents.[21] Dextroamphetamine may produce tachyphylaxis requiring dose increases. Therefore, methylphenidate is the psychostimulant of choice.

Antidepressants

The following issues are generally evaluated when choosing an antidepressant:[8,22]

- side-effect profile
- existing medical problems (drug-disease interactions)
- drug-drug interactions
- nature of depressive symptoms
- past response to specific antidepressive agents

Selective Serotonin Reuptake Inhibitors

Selective serotonin reuptake inhibitors (SSRIs) have many fewer anticholinergic side effects than tricyclic antidepressants and are less sedating. Urinary retention and memory impairment are usually not associated with their use. The SSRIs rarely impair cardiac conduction or cause orthostatic hypotension; however, increased intestinal motility (resulting in diarrhea), nausea, vomiting, insomnia, restlessness, anxiety, headaches, and sexual dysfunction are common side effects. Because the SSRIs have a more favorable adverse effect profile, Massie and Popkin have selected them as first-line antidepressants.[7]

The major differences among the SSRIs are half-life and drug interactions. Fluoxetine and its active metabolite have a half-life of several days limiting its utility in terminally ill patients. Sertraline, paroxetine, and citalopram have half-lives of approximately one day, and fluvoxamine's half-life is only 15 hours. There are no major clinical distinctions between the SSRIs. Citalopram may have the advantage of fewer drug interactions than the other SSRIs. They are structurally dissimilar, and patients who fail one SSRI may respond to another.

Tricyclic Antidepressants

Patients who need additional sedation, anxiolysis, and analgesia may benefit from a tricyclic antidepressant (TCA). However, TCAs have profound anticholinergic, α_1-adrenoreceptor antagonistic, and antihistaminic effects. Slowed gastrointestinal tract and genitourinary tract motility, delirium, tachycardia, postural hypotension, dizziness, and/or sedation are common adverse effects. If any of these effects is intolerable or unacceptable, a different antidepressant agent should be considered. TCAs can cause cardiac conduction abnormalities. Caution is warranted in patients with an underlying conduction defect and in patients on concomitant drug therapy that affects ventricular impulse conduction.[16,23]

In general, secondary amines cause fewer anticholinergic and cardiovascular effects and less sedation than the tertiary amines. Nortriptyline and desipramine, both secondary amines, are the safest and best tolerated. Amitriptyline, doxepin, and trimipramine are the most sedating TCAs, and may be most useful in agitated patients or patients who have difficulty sleeping. They also have the strongest anticholinergic and orthostatic effects.[16,19,23]

Cancer patients have demonstrated response to TCAs at lower doses than those used to treat healthy patients. Why this occurs is unknown. Patients should start at one-third the anticipated therapeutic dose and increase to the target dose one to two weeks. This schedule will help to minimize adverse effects and allow continued titration to a therapeutic response. Depressive symptoms generally respond to treatment in four weeks. If no benefit is gained before the onset of unacceptable adverse effects, alternative antidepressive agents should be considered.

Both TCAs and SSRIs can be administered as oral liquids and rectal suppositories. Amitriptyline, imipramine, and clomipramine suppositories can be compounded easily.[24,25] Fluoxetine, nortriptyline, and doxepin are available in liquid formulations

Other Antidepressant Agents

Bupropion affects noradrenergic and dopaminergic neurotransmitter systems. It may be most appropriately used in depressed patients who are withdrawn, anhedonic, inattentive, or have psychomotor retardation due to its "activating" effect. Side effects of bupropion are generally due to adrenergic excess, e.g., agitation and insomnia. It is best to avoid bupropion in patients with a seizure history or CNS tumor involvement. Bupropion is a reasonable second line agent in patients who fail SSRI therapy or in whom SSRIs are contraindicated.

Trazodone and nefazodone are structurally similar. Both inhibit serotonin reuptake and block postsynaptic serotonin 5-HT$_2$ receptors. Trazodone is also an antagonist of postsynaptic alpha adrenergic receptors. It causes significant sedation, so the role of trazodone in palliative care may best be in the treatment of insomnia. Patients must be informed of the possibility that priapism may occur and what to do if it does.

There is little information regarding the use of nefazodone in palliative care patients; most review articles discuss only trazodone. Nefazodone has a more favorable side effect profile than trazodone. No reports have been made of nefazodone-induced priapism, and it does not cause as much sedation as trazodone. Nefazodone may be a reasonable alternative in patients with agitated depression.[7,19]

Venlafaxine and mirtazapine act by affecting several neurotransmitter systems and may be effective agents in patients who fail to respond to serotonin modulation alone. Venlafaxine is well tolerated, but patients taking it should be monitored for hypertension. Mirtazapine is highly sedating and may cause weight gain. Bedtime dosing may allow exploitation of the former side effect. It is reasonable to assume that terminally ill patients will respond favorably to venlafaxine and mirtazapine; however, no data are available comparing them to other antidepressant agents in palliative care.

Maprotiline and amoxapine have both been associated with an increase in seizure propensity. In addition, amoxapine's dopamine blocking effect may cause extrapyramidal side effects especially when other dopaminergic agents are used. Consequently, maprotiline and amoxapine are rarely used in palliative care.

Monoamine oxidase inhibitors (MAOIs) are reserved as last line alternatives in the general psychiatric population as well as in the terminally ill population. They cannot be used in patients receiving sympathomimetic agents, opioids, psychostimulants, or chemotherapy. In addition, patients have to watch their diet closely avoiding

TABLE 2. System-Based Pharmacotherapy for Managing Depression in Palliative Care*

Target Symptoms	Primary Agent	Alternatives	AWP per Month of Therapy	Medications to Avoid
Short life expectancy and/or need for immediate relief	**methylphenidate (Ritalin)** Initial: 2.5 mg PO QAM or 2.5 mg PO 8AM & Noon Range: 5-30 mg	**dextroamphetamine (Dexedrine)** Initial: 2.5 mg PO QAM or 2.5 mg PO 8AM & N. Range: 5-30 mg **pemoline (Cylert)** Initial: 18.75 mg PO QAM or 18.75 mg PO 8AM & N. Range: 37.5-150 mg	methylphenidate 5 mg PO BID $16.86 dextroamphetamine 5 mg PO BID $10.55 pemoline 37.5 mg PO BID $70.99	
Anhedonia withdrawal, Psychomotor retardation	**bupropion (Wellbutrin)** Initial: 50 mg PO QD Range: 150-300 mg **methylphenidate (Ritalin)** Initial: 2.5 mg PO QAM or 2.5 mg PO 8AM & Noon Range: 5-30 mg	**dextroamphetamine (Dexedrine)** Initial: 2.5 mg PO QAM or 2.5 mg PO 8AM & Noon Range: 5-30 mg **pemoline (Cylert)** Initial: 18.75 mg PO QAM or 18.75 mg PO 8AM & Noon Range: 37.5-150 mg	bupropion 100 mg PO QD $24.89 methylphenidate 5 mg PO BID $16.86 dextroamphetamine 5 mg PO BID $10.55p pemoline 37.5 mg PO BID $70.99	
Anorexia	**desipramine (Norpramin))** Initial: 12.5-25 mg PO HS Range: 75-100 mg **nortriptyline (Aventlyl, Pamelor)** Initial: 10-25 mg PO HS Range: 25-100 mg	**amitriptyline (Elavil)** Initial: 10-25 mg PO HS Range: 50-100 mg **doxepin (Sinequan, Adapin)** Initial: 25 mg PO HS Range: 75-100 mg **mirtazapine (Remeron)** Initial: 15 mg PO QD Range: 15-45 mg	desipramine 75 mg PO HS $16.95 nortriptyline 25 mg PO HS $22.31 amitriptyline 50 mg PO HS $ 3.36 doxepin 75 mg PO HS $ 9.75 mirtazapine 15 mg PO QD $59.40	SSRI's may cause problems initially

Insomnia and/or agitation	**Amitriptyline (Elavil)** Initial: 10-25 mg PO HS Range: 50-100 mg **doxepin (Sinequan, Adapin)** Initial: 25 mg PO HS Range: 75-100 mg	**desipramine (Norpramin)** Initial: 12.5-25 mg PO HS Range: 75-100 mg **nortriptyline (Aventyl, Pamelor)** Initial: 10-25 mg PO HS Range: 25-100 mg **trazodone (Deseryl)** Initial: 50 mg PO HS Range: 150-300 mg **nefazodone (Serzone)** Initial: 100 mg PO HS Range: 200-500 mg	amitriptyline 50 mg PO HS $ 3.36 doxepin 75 mg PO HS $ 9.75 desipramine 75 mg PO HS $16.95 nortriptyline 25 mg PO HS $22.31 trazodone 150 mg PO HS $26.78 nefazodone 200 mg PO HS $14.96	TCA's trazodone nefazodone
Somnolence, excessive sedation	**citalopram (Celexa)** Initial: 10 mg PO QD Rarge: 20-40 mg **fluoxetine (Prosac)** Initial: 10 mg PO QD Range: 20-40 mg **paroxetine (Paxil)** Initial: 15 mg PO QD Range: 30-60 mg	**sertraline (Zoloft)** Initial: 25 mg PO QD Range: 50-100 mg **bupropion (Wellbutrin)** Initial: 50 mg PO QD Range: 150-300 mg **venlafaxine (Effexor)** Initial: 18.75 mg PO QD Range: 75-375 mg	citalopram 20 mg PO QD $57.96 fluoxetine 20 mg PO QD $67.36 paroxetine 20 mg PO QD $56.97 sertraline 50 mg PO QD $52.87 bupropion 100 mg PO QD $24.89 venlafaxine 37.5 mg PO BID $58.99	TCA's trazodone nefazodone
Seizure potential	**citalopram (Remeron)** Initial: 10 mg PO QD Range: 20-40 mg flucuetine **(Prozac)** Initial: 10 mg PO QD Range: 20-40 mg **paroxetine (Paxil)** Initial: 10 mg PO QD Range: 20-40 mg **sertraline (Zoloft)** Initial: 25 mg PO QD Range: 50-200 mg	**trazodone (Desyrel)** Initial: 50 mg PO HS Range: 150-300 mg **venlafaxine (Effexor)** Initial: 18.75 mg PO QD Range: 75-375 mg	citalopram 20 mg PO QD $57.96 fluoxetine 20 mg PO QD $67.36 paroxetine 20 mg PO QD $56.97 sertraline 50 mg PO QD $52.87 trazodone 150 mg PO HS $26.78 venlafaxine 37.5 mg PO BID $58.99	TCAs bupropion amoxapine maprotiline
Suicidal ideation				TCAs, amoxapine maprotiline

* Evaluate patient in terms of *target symptoms* found in Table 2 and in terms of *pharmacotherapeutic considerations* in Table 3. Make drug selection. If no symptoms or issues are identified, then consider starting treatment with an SSRI. See treatment algorithm.

TABLE 3. Pharmacotherapeutic Considerations for the Management of Depression in Palliative Care Patients (Interactions represent relative and absolute contraindications; evaluate on a case by case basis.)

Therapeutic Alternatives	Side Effect Profile	Drug-Disease Interactions	Drug-Drug Interactions	Nature of Depressive Symptoms
Tricyclic Antidepressants Secondary Amines desipramine (Norpramin) nortriptyline (Aventyl, Pamelor) protriptyline (Vivactyl)	Anticholinergic effects, sedation, orthostatic hypotension, seizures, conduction abnormalities	recent myocardial infarction, conduction problems, history of or suspected seizure disorder, urinary retention, angle-closure glaucoma, hyperthyroidism, impaired cognition, cirrhosis	CYP2D6 inhibitors and inducers Monoamine Oxidase Inhibitors Drugs that prolong QTc interval: cisapride, erythromycin, class I and III antiarrhythmics, etc.	nortriptyline and desipramine least anticholinergic and cardiovascular side effects (best tolerated) amitriptyline, trimipramine, and doxepin: depression with agitation and/or insomnia
Tricyclic Antidepressants Tertiary Amines amitriptyline (Elavil) doxepin (Sinequan, Adapin) imipramine (Tofranil) trimipramine (Surmontil)	Same side effects with greater intensity as secondary amine TCAs	same as secondary amine TCAs	same as secondary amine TCAs	same as secondary amine TCAs
Selective Serotonin Reuptake Inhibitor Antidepressants citalopram (Celexa) fluoxetine (Prozac) fluvoxamine (Fluvox) paroxetine (Paxil) sertraline	Nausea, vomiting, diarrhea, nervousness, agitation, anxiety, headache, insomnia, fatigue, rash	cirrhosis, impaired cognition, bipolar disorder (activation of mania)	monoamine oxidase inhibitors, tryptophan, warfarin, cimetidine, phenobarbital, phenytoin, drugs metabolized by CYP2D6, 3A4, 2D5, diazepam, digoxin, beta blockers, theophylline	cachectic or anorexic: GI side effects may be problematic initially
amoxapine (Asendin)	Seizure, extrapyramidal effects, sedation, anticholinergic effects	urinary retention, angle-closure glaucoma, recent myocardial infarction, cardiovascular disorders	monoamine oxidase inhibitors, tricyclic antidepressants, cimetidine	seizure risk/history, concomitant dopaminergic medications, suicidal ideation: dangerous in overdose, may promote seizure activity, EPS adverse effects

Drug	Side effects	Contraindications / Precautions	Drug interactions	Notes
bupropion (Wellbutrin)	Seizure, nausea, dizziness, tremor, insomnia, vomiting, constipation, skin reactions	History of or suspected seizure disorder, head trauma, or CNS tumor; neuropsychiatric phenomena; hepatic dysfunction	CYP2B6 inducers and inhibitors (phenytoin, phenobarbital, carbamazepine, cimetidine)	psychomotor retardation, withdrawal, anhedonia: bupropion may exhibit "activating" effect; Seizure risk/history: may lower seizure threshold
maprotiline (Ludiomil)	Seizure, sedation, mild anticholinergic effects, rash	History of or suspected seizure disorder, myocardial infarction, cardiovascular disease, conduction defects, dysrhythmias, stroke, hyperthyroidism	monoamine oxidase inhibitors, anticholinergic agents, sympathomimetic agents, guanethidine, phenothiazines, cimetidine	Seizure risk/history, suicidal ideation: dangerous in overdose, may promote seizure activity
mirtazapine (Remeron)	Somnolence, increased appetite, dizziness dry mouth, constipation, increased cholesterol and triglycerides	Cirrhosis, bipolar disorder (may induce mania)	benzodiazepines (motor function impairment); drugs metabolized by CYP 2D6, 1A2, 3A4 (no studies conducted–use with caution)	Cachectic pt. or poor appetite: may increase appetite and promote weight gain
nefazodone (Serzone)	Lightheadedness, dizziness, orthostatic hypotension, somnolence, dry mouth, nausea, asthenia	Effects on patients with cardiovascular disease and conduction abnormalities not known.	Monoamine oxidase inhibitors, highly protein bound drugs, haloperidol CYP3A4 substrates (triazolam, alprazolam, cisapride), digoxin, popranolol	Insomnia, agitation: beneficial sedating effect
trazodone (Desyrel)	Sedation, dysrhythmias, priapism	Recent myocardial infarction, history of cardiac disease	phenytoin, monoamine oxidase inhibitors, warfarin	Insomnia, agitation: beneficial sedating effect
venlafaxine (Effexor)	Hypertension, nausea, mild anticholinergic effects, anorexia	Recent myocardial infarction, unstable heart disease, renal impairment, cirrhosis	highly protein bound drugs, monoamine oxidase inhibitors, cimetidine, drugs that inhibit CYP2D6	

TABLE 3 (continued)

Therapeutic Alternatives	Side Effect Profile	Drug-Disease Interactions	Drug-Drug Interactions	Nature of Depressive Symptoms
MAOI phenelzine (Nardil) tranylcypromine (Parnate)	Hypertensive crisis, postural hypotension, anticholinergic effects,	Cardiovascular disorders, pheochromocytoma, hyperthyroidism, anxiety/agitation, history or risk of seizure disorder	tyramine, opioids,\ bupropion, SSRI's, buspirone, sympathomimetics (amphetamines, pseudoephedrine), guanethidine, methyldopa, reserpine, dopamine, levodopa, tryptophan, meperidine, dextromethorphan	
Stimulants dextroamphetamine (Dexedrine) methylphenidate (Ritalin) pemoline (Cylert)	Nervousness, insomnia,	Arteriosclerosis,	monoamine oxidase inhibitors	Short life expectancy, need for monitoring

86

tyramine containing foods. Consequently, their utility as pharmacotherapy for terminally ill patients is extremely limited.

CONCLUSION

Depression often is not viewed as a problem in palliative care patients, and it may be difficult to identify. When a diagnosis has been made, very little evidence is available for physicians to consider when evaluating treatment options. Methylphenidate can be a useful mood elevator in terminally ill patients. The onset is rapid, but patients should be monitored for excessive stimulation and other adverse effects. TCAs and SSRIs have been widely used, and SSRIs are generally considered the antidepressants of choice. It is unclear how the newer, miscellaneous antidepressant agents should be used in this patient population. Pharmacokinetic and pharmacodynamic considerations can provide clues to appropriate use, but comparative clinical trials are needed to delineate how antidepressive agents compare in terms of efficacy and safety when used to treat depression in palliative care patient

SOME OPEN RESEARCH QUESTIONS

1. How does the depression of a terminally ill patient differ from the depression of a medically ill patient, a cancer patient, and a healthy person?
2. How should the pharmacologic intervention change to address the needs of the terminally ill patient, i.e., target specific receptors or neurotransmitters, onset of action, ADE profile, interaction profile?
3. What is the role of the psychostimulants?

REFERENCES

1. Goldberg RJ. Management of depression in the patient with advanced cancer. JAMA. 1981;246:373-6.

2. Barraclough J. ABC of palliative care: depression, anxiety, and confusion. BMJ. 1997;315:1365-8.

3. Breitbart W. Identifying patients at risk for, and treatment of major psychiatric complications of cancer. Support Care Cancer. 1995;3:45-60.

4. Minagawa H, Uchitomi Y, Yamawaki S, Ishitani K. Psychiatric morbidity in terminally ill cancer patients. Cancer. 1996;78:1131-7.

5. Chochinov HM, Wilson KG, Enns M, Landers S. Prevalence of depression in the terminally ill: effects of diagnostic criteria and symptom threshold judgments. Am J Psychiatry. 1994;151:537-40.

6. Andrykowski MA, Curran SL, Lightner R. Off-treatment fatigue in breast cancer survivors: a controlled comparison. J Behavior Med. 1998;21:1-17.

7. Massie JM, Popkin MK. Depressive disorders. In: Holland JC, ed. Psycho-oncology. New York: Oxford University Press; 1998:518-40.

8. Breitbart W, Passik SD. Psychiatric aspects of palliative care. In: Doyle D, Hanks GWC, MacDonald N, eds. Oxford Textbook of Palliative Medicine. New York: Oxford University Press; 1993:609-26.

9. Breitbart W, Jacobsen PB. Psychiatric symptom management in terminal care. Clin Geriatr Med. 1996;12:329-347.

10. Anon. Some drugs that cause psychiatric symptoms. Med Lett. 1998;40:20-4.

11. Chochinov HM, Wilson KG, Enns M, Lander S. "Are you depressed?" Screening for depression in the terminally ill. Am. J. Psychiatry. 1997;154:674-6.

12. Zigmond AS, Snaith RP. The Hospital Anxiety and Depression Scale. Acta Psychiatr Scand. 1983;67:361-70.

13. Cramond WA. Psychotherapy of the dying patient. BMJ. 1970;3:389-93.

14. Wood BC, Mynors-Wallis LM. Problem-solving therapy in palliative care. Palliat Med. 1997;11:49-54.

15. Bidder TG. Electroconvulsive therapy in the medically ill patient. Psychiatric Clinics of North America. 1981;4:391-405.

16. Breitbart W, Jacobsen PB. Psychiatric symptom management in terminal care. Clin Geritr Med. 1996;12:329-47.

17. Breitbart W, Bruera E, Chochinov H, Lynch M. Neuropsychiatric syndromes and psychological symptoms in patients with advanced cancer. J Pain Symptom Manage. 1995;10:131-41.

18. Kinzel T. Relief of emotional symptoms in elderly patients with terminal cancer. Geriatrics. 1988;43:61-5,68.

19. Roth AJ, Breitbart W. Psychiatric emergencies in terminally ill cancer patients. Hematol Oncol Clin North Am. 1996;10:235-59.

20. Holmes VF. Medical use of psychostimulants: an overview. Int J Psychiatry Med. 1995;25:1-19.

21. Yee JD, Berde CB. Dextroamphetamine or methylphenidate as adjuvants to opioid analgesia for adolescents with cancer. J Pain Symptom Manage. 1994;9:122-5.

22. Roth AJ, Breitbart W. Psychiatric emergencies in terminally ill cancer patients. Pain and Palliat Care. 1996;10:235-59.

23. Rudorfer MV, Manji HK, Potter WZ. Comparative tolerability profiles of the newer versus older antidepressants. Drug Saf. 1994;10:18-46.

24. Chaumeil JC, Khoury JM, Zuber M, et al. Formulation of suppositories containing imipramine and clomipramine chlorhydrates. Drug Dev Indust Pharm. 1988;14:2225-39.

25. Adams F. Amitriptyline suppositories. N Engl J Med. 1982;306:996.

26. Cohen SR. Phototherapy In the treatment of depression in the terminally ill. Symptom Manage. 1994;9:534-6.

27. Johnston B. Relief of mixed anxiety-depression in terminal cancer patients: effect of thioridazine. New York State J Med. 1972;73:2315-17.

28. Maisami M, Sohmer BH, Coyle JT. Combined use of tricyclic antidepressants and neuroleptics in the management of terminally ill children: a report on three cases. J Amer Academy Child Psychiatry. 1985;24:487-9.

29. Sheehan MK, Janicak PG, Dowd S. The role of psychopharmacotherapy in the dying patient. Psychiatric Annals. 1994;24:98-103.

30. Malitz S, Goldstein E. Psychotherapy and pharmacotherapy in a dying patient: report of a supervised case. J Thanatol. 1972;2:744-56.

31. Macleod AD. Methylphenidate in terminal depression. J Pain Symptom Manage. 1998;16:193-8.

32. Breitbart W, Mermelstein H. Pemoline: an alternative psychostimulant for the management of depressive disorders in cancer patients. Psychosomatics. 1992;33:352-6.

Diarrhea in Palliative Care Patients

M. Christina Beckwith

SUMMARY. Diarrhea in palliative care patients may be acute or chronic and may be due to infection or overuse of laxatives. Potential causes of diarrhea are discussed. Studies of drug therapy in the management of diarrhea in advanced disease patients are summarized. Evaluation instruments that have been used to assess this symptom are described. Some open research questions are listed. Four treatment algorithms, evidence tables and drug therapy tables which include drug costs are presented. *[Article copies available for a fee from The Haworth Document Delivery Service: 1-800-342-9678. E-mail address: getinfo@ haworthpressinc.com <Website: http://www.haworthpressinc.com>]*

KEYWORDS. Diarrhea, bowels, fecal impaction, palliative care, terminal care, dying, supportive care, drug therapy, non-pharmacological therapy, etiology, evidence, costs, algorithm, aspirin, cholestyramine, octreotide, bismuth subsalicylate, codeine, cyproheptadine, diphenoxylate, loperamide, kaolin, pectin, lipase, opium, opioids, psyllium

M. Christina Beckwith, PharmD, is Drug Information Specialist, Department of Pharmacy Services, University Hospitals and Clinics, University of Utah, Salt Lake City, UT.

Address correspondence to: Arthur G. Lipman, PharmD, College of Pharmacy and Pain Management Center, 30 S 2000 E RM 258, University of Utah Health Sciences Center, Salt Lake City, UT 84112-5820 (E-mail: alipman@pharm.utah.edu).

[Haworth co-indexing entry note]: "Diarrhea in Palliative Care Patients." Beckwith, M. Chirstina. Co-published simultaneously in *Journal of Pharmaceutical Care in Pain & Symptom Control* (Pharmaceutical Products Press, an imprint of The Haworth Press, Inc.) Vol. 7, No. 4, 1999, pp. 91-108; and: *Evidence Based Symptom Control in Palliative Care: Systematic Reviews and Validated Clinical Practice Guidelines for 15 Common Problems in Patients with Life Limiting Disease* (ed: Arthur G. Lipman, Kenneth C. Jackson II, and Linda S. Tyler) Pharmaceutical Products Press, an imprint of The Haworth Press, Inc., 2000, pp. 91-108. Single or multiple copies of this article are available for a fee from The Haworth Document Delivery Service [1-800-342-9678, 9:00 a.m. - 5:00 p.m. (EST). E-mail address: getinfo@haworthpressinc. com].

Algorithm for Managing Diarrhea: Acute Diarrhea

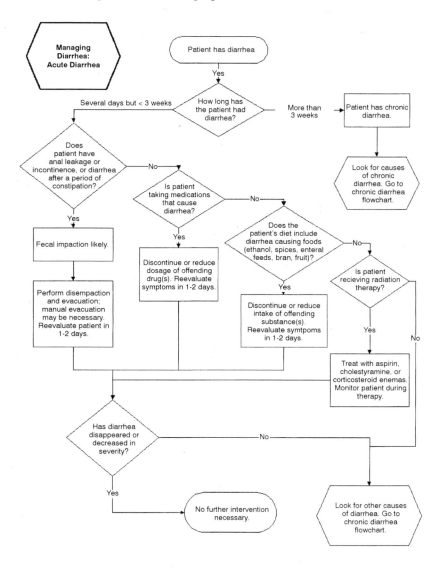

Algorithm for Managing Diarrhea: Chronic Diarrhea

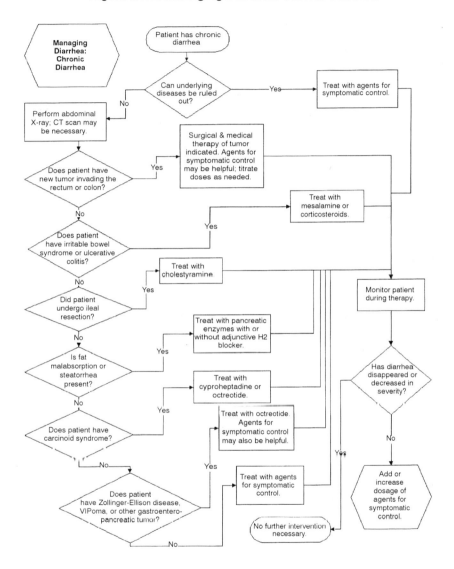

Algorithm for Managing Diarrhea: Infectious Causes

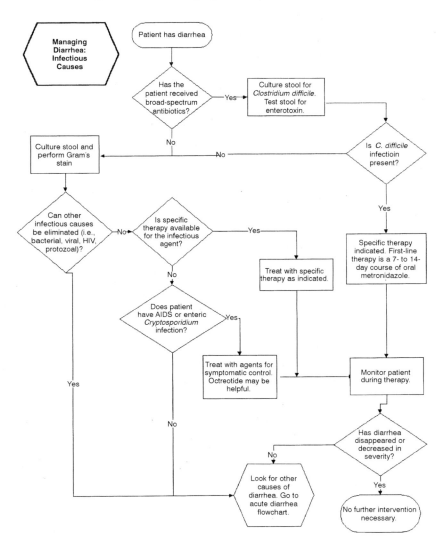

Algorithm for Managing Diarrhea: Induced by Laxatives

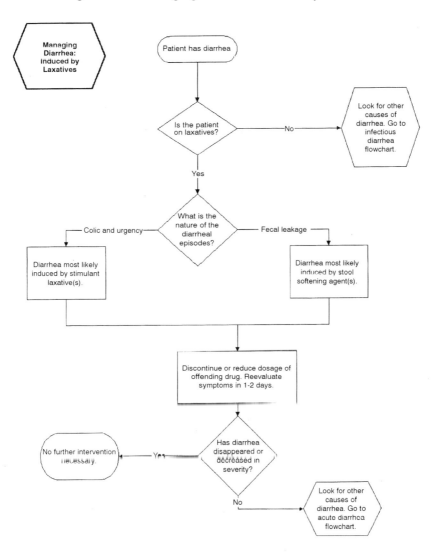

Diarrhea occurs in about 6% of terminally ill cancer patients,[1] 5% to 10% of hospice patients,[2,3] and 27% to 50% of AIDS patients.[4,5] Several causes and consequences of diarrhea in palliative care have been described.[1-4] In one case series of 120 cancer patients, diarrhea was reported to be unrelated to severity of other symptoms, but caused significant distress in 10% of patients.[6] Few clinical trials have evaluated the efficacy of medications for diarrhea in this population. Table 1 summarizes the evidence from available trials for managing diarrhea with pharmacologic interventions.

Diarrhea is defined as increased frequency and liquidity of feces,[7] usually interpreted as passage of more than 3 unformed stools within a 24-hour period.[4] Diarrhea may refer to a single loose stool, fecal incontinence, or frequent passage of small stools of normal or hard consistency. Diarrhea is acute in most cases and lasts only a few days. Episodes persisting longer than 3 weeks are considered chronic and are usually caused by organic disease.[4] Malnutrition, dehydration, electrolyte depletion, and pressure sore formation may be worsened by diarrhea.[3]

EVALUATE THE CAUSES OF DIARRHEA

Evaluate each patient with diarrhea to identify potential causes. Careful evaluation of patient history and rectal examination are necessary to guide selection of appropriate therapy. The most common causes of diarrhea in palliative care patients are laxative overuse[3] and leakage around a fecal impaction.[1,2] Anal leakage may occur following surgical or pathological injury to the anal sphincter.[1] Diarrhea may occur secondary to underlying disease in patients with AIDS or with metastases invading the colon or rectum.[1-3] Rarely, endocrine tumors cause secretory diarrhea.[4] Absence of fecal masses on abdominal palpation excludes fecal impaction in most cases although abdominal radiography may sometimes be required.[3,4] Stool culture and Gram stain should be performed when the feces contains blood or white blood cells and in patients with AIDS[3,5] or a history of recent travel to warm climates.[4] Pale, fatty, smelly stool suggests steatorrhea and fat malabsorption. Persistent, watery diarrhea with an anion gap above 50 mmol/L suggests osmotic diarrhea due to unabsorbed solute, e.g., sorbitol, while an anion gap below 50 mmol/L suggests secretory diarrhea.[4]

TREAT THE UNDERLYING CAUSE WHEN POSSIBLE

When possible, the underlying cause of the symptom should be treated. Frequent treatable causes of diarrhea include:[1 5,8]

- laxative overuse
- fecal impaction
- bacterial infection;
    > likely pathogens include *Salmonella* species, *Shigella* species, and *Campylobacter. Mycobacterium avium-intracellulare* is another possible cause of diarrhea in AIDS patients.

- viral infection; in AIDS patients;
    > likely pathogens include cytomegalovirus, adenovirus, and human immunodeficiency virus (HIV) itself. Rotavirus and Norwalk-type virus are other possible pathogens in palliative care patients. Of these, specific treatment is available only for cytomegalovirus infection.

- enteric protozoal infections may occur in AIDS patients;
    > pathogens include *Cryptosporidium, Microsporidium, Giardia, Isospora*, or *Cyanobacterium*-like bodies. Avoid broad-spectrum antibiotic therapy. Use narrow spectrum antimicrobials whenever possible. *Clostridium difficile* infection may cause diarrhea in patients receiving antibiotics. Some clinicians suggest candidal overgrowth may also be a culprit.

- radiation-induced gastrointestinal (GI) damage;
    > incidence of diarrhea is highest during the second and third weeks of radiation to the abdomen or pelvis.

- bile salt diarrhea secondary to ileal resection and subsequent reduced bile acid reabsorption
- malabsorption and steatorrhea secondary to decreased pancreatic function
- Zollinger-Ellison disease
- vasoactive intestinal peptide tumor (VIPoma)
- carcinoid syndrome
- irritable bowel syndrome or ulcerative colitis
- enteral feeding
- anxiety

IMPLEMENT SUPPORTIVE THERAPY

Many non-pharmacologic measures can be implemented to treat diarrhea and support the patient during the diarrheal episode. These may include the following:[1-4,8-10]

- decrease dietary intake of solid matter, including bran and fruit.
- reduce rate or osmolarity of enteral nutrition formula, if applicable
- encourage oral rehydration with glucose and electrolyte solutions, if possible. Intravenous rehydration may be necessary
- in severe cases decrease intake of alcohol and hot spices
- decrease milk intake since bacterial causes of diarrhea may cause transient lactase deficiency
- discontinue or reduce dosage of offending medications, including
  - antihypertensives, including guanethidine and propranolol
  - retrovirals, including lamivudine and zidovudine
  - some chemotherapeutic agents, including fluorouracil and mitomycin
  - cholinergic agents such as bethanechol, neostigmine, and pyridostigmine
  - laxatives
  - magnesium-containing antacids and magnesium supplements
  - methylxanthines, including caffeine and theophylline
  - some non-steroidal anti-inflammatory drugs (NSAIDS), including diclofenac, indomethacin, meclofenamate, mefenamic acid, nabumetone
  - potassium supplements
  - prokinetic agents, including cisapride and metoclopramide
  - prostaglandins including carboprost, dinoprostone, and misoprostol
  - quinidine
  - sorbitol

- thiazide diuretics, e.g., chlorothiazide, chlorthalidone, hydrochlorothiazide

- clean the perianal area frequently to prevent skin breakdown
- apply barrier creams or zinc oxide paste may provide increased protection
- disempact and manually evacuate stool in patients with fecal impaction.

CONCLUSION

Diarrhea occurs in 6% of terminal cancer patients, 5% to 10% of hospice patients,[2,3] and 27% to 50% of AIDS patients.[5] Diarrhea may contribute to malnutrition, dehydration, electrolyte depletion, and formation of pressure sores.[3] Thorough patient history and evaluation are the key to selecting appropriate therapy for the underlying cause of diarrhea. Both non-pharmacologic and pharmacologic methods may be used for symptomatic control of diarrhea. Adjunctive therapy is aimed at preventing dehydration and replacing electrolytes.

SOME OPEN RESEARCH QUESTIONS

1. How much of a problem are adverse effects with these drugs when used to treat diarrhea?
2. What is the usefulness of combination therapy?
3. Is antidiarrheal drug therapy indicated for patients with documented infectious cause of diarrhea?
4. Does antidiarrheal drug therapy decrease with chronic maintenance therapy (i.e., octreotide in AIDS patients with refractory diarrhea or *Cryptosporidium* infection).

TABLE 1. Drug Therapy for Managing Diarrhea in Palliative Care–Evidence Tables

Reference	Study Design	n	Intervention	Results	Level of Evidence	Comments
Aspirin						
Mennie et al. (1975)[12]	Randomized, double-blind, placebo-controlled	28	Uterine cancer patients with diarrhea secondary to radiation therapy received aspirin 972 mg PO QID or vehicle PO QID for 72 hours. Patients asked not to take any other antidiarrheals.	Number of bowel movements/day decreased in 11/14 aspirin patients and in 3/14 vehicle patients (p < 0.004). Compared with vehicle, more patients reported relief of abdominal pain (p < 0.001) and flatulence (p < 0.03) with aspirin.	II	Diarrhea recurred following study discontinuation in 7/11 aspirin-treated patients responding to therapy.
Cholestyramine (Questran, Prevalite)						
Condon et al. (1978)[11]	Descriptive	1	Bladder cancer patient with radiation-induced diarrhea given cholestyramine 4 g PO every 6 hours and 4 g PO at night for 3 days. Patient had been treated with opiates, diphenoxylate/atropine, and kaolin with inadequate response. Antidiarrheals stopped 3 days prior to cholestyramine.	Averge number of stools per day decreased from 18.0 at baseline to 2.3 during cholestyramine therapy. Daily fecal weight decreased (178.2 g at baseline) to 57.3 g with cholestyramine although fecal dry weight remained similar at baseline (14.9 g/day) and during treatment (15.5 g/day).	V	None.
Octreotide (Sandostatin)						
Brabant et al. (1986)[14]	Descriptive	5	Patients with carcinoid syndrome (n = 4) and VIPoma (n = 1) received octreotide 50 mcg SC BID to QID (up to 500 mcg SC QID in 1 patient) for 3 to 52 weeks.	Diarrheal episodes and abdominal cramping decreased in patients with these symptoms before therapy (n = 4 and n = 3, respectively). In one carcinoid patient, slight decrease in diarrheal episodes/day (from 4-6 to 4) with doses up to 500 mc SC QID.	V	None.

Cello et al. (1991)[18]	Prospective, open-label, multicenter	51	HIV-infected patients with refractory diarrhea given octreotide 50 mcg SC every 8 hours. If stool volume 250 mL/day, dose increased every 48 hours to 100, 250, or 500 mcg SC TID. After 14 days of therapy, patients discharged on lowest effective dose and tapered off after 7 days. Response to therapy considered complete if stool volume < 250 mL/day; partial response if stool volume > 250 mL/day but reduced 50% from baseline. Refractory diarrhea defined as 500 mL/day liquid stool for 4 weeks despite 2 weeks of antidiarrheal drugs.	Response occurred in 41.2% (21/51) of patients: complete response in 7/21 and partial response in 14/21. Octreotide 100, 200, and 500 mcg SC TID significantly reduced stool volume and frequency; no effect with 50 mcg dose. Daily number of stools decreased from 6.5 ± 0.5 at baseline to 3.8 ± 0.4 on Day 14 ($p < 0.01$) and $3.810.3$ on Day 21 ($p = .0001$). Daily stool volume also decreased, from 1604 ± 180 mL at baseline to 1084 ± 162 mL on Day 14 ($p < 0.001$).	IV	Stool frequency returned to 4.8 ± 0.6 mL/day ($p > 0.05$ vs. baseline) on Day 28 after octreotide discontinuation. Nonresponders more likely than responders to have identifiable pathogens in the stool (70% vs. 33% respectively, $p < 0.01$). No difference between nonresponders and responders in incidence of cryptosporidium infection (33% vs. 24%, $p > .05$).
Cictet et al. (1989)[25]	Descriptive	4	AIDS patients with cryptosporidial diarrhea given octreotide SC every 8 hours in doses escalating from 50 mcg to 50C mcg. Therapy continued with minimal effective dose for 15 days for complete responders and indefinitely for partial responders. Partial response defined as >50% reduction in symptoms and number of stools/day; complete response as total disappearance of diarrhea.	Complete and partial responses achieved in 1/4 patients (25%) each. No recurrence of diarrhea for 9 months in the complete responder. Diarrhea recurred within 1 month in the partial responder, despite continued therapy. None.	V	

TABLE 1 (continued)

Reference	Study Design	n	Intervention	Results	Level of Evidence	Comments
Cook et al. (1988)[24]	Descriptive	1	AIDS patient with cryptosporidial diarrhea refractory to conventional antidiarrheals given octreotide 100, 200, and 300 mcg SC TID.	Daily stool volume decreased from 2.5-3.2 L at baseline to 0.4-1.1 L during therapy with 200-300 mcg SC TID. Stool frequency decreased from 10-22/day to 2-6/day with octreotide 200-300 mcg SC TID. Octreotide 100 mcg SC TID decreased stool volume and frequency for a short time only then increasing doses were required.	V	Patient maintained on octreotide 300 mcg SC TID for 8 months without diarrhea, eating a normal diet.
Fanning et al. (1991)[17]	Prospective, open-label, dose-finding	17	AIDS patients with diarrhea refractory to 1 week of antidiarrheals given octreotide 50 mcg SC TID. If diarrhea not controlled, dose increased every 48 hours to 100, 250, or 500 mcg SC TID. Once controlled, continued same dose for 2 weeks. Response defined as 3 stools/day and/or 50% reduction in daily stool volume. Diarrhea defined as > 3 unformed bowel movements daily and/or stool volume of 1 L/day. Total duration of diarrhea was >1 month in all patients.	45% (5/11) of evaluable patients had good response to octreotide doses of 50 mcg SC TID (n = 2), 100 mcg SC TID (n = 2), and 250 mcg SC TID (n = 1). Moderate response to 250 mcg SC TID in 9% (1/11) of patients, evidenced by a slight decrease in stool volume. Compared with baseline, number of bowel movements daily decreased with octreotide in the responders (p = 0.0431).	IV	After octreotide discontinued, number of bowel movements increased significantly (p = 0.0431 vs. treatment period). The 5 responders were maintained on octreotide after the study; 60% (3/5) on the original dose. The other two required dosage increases but discontinued therapy within 3-12 months due to adverse effects (n = 1) or loss of efficacy (n = 1). Only 1/3 patients (33%) with enteric *Cryptosporidium* had a good response.
Geelhoed et al. (1986)[13]	Descriptive	2	Patients with severe diarrhea given octreotide 100 mcg SC BID for 2 months, then 250 mcg SC BID for 1-2 months. Diarrhea caused by Zollinger-Ellison disease and medullary thyroid carcinoma, in 1 patient each. Patients continued therapy for underlying disease.	Subjective improvement in both patients (no statistical analysis). Patient with Zollinger-Ellison disease had a dose-related decrease in tumor markers and needed lower doses of other agents. No change in tumor markers seen in patient with medullary thyroid carcinoma.	V	None.

Study	Type	N	Description	Results	Level	Outcome
Katz et al. (1988)[23]	Descriptive	1	AIDS patient with cryptosporidial diarrhea refractory to other agents given octreotide 1800-2400 mcg/day by continuous IV infusion for > 9 months.	Daily stool volume decreased from 6 L at baseline to 3 L on day 10 of therapy.	V	Diarrhea and abdominal cramping recurred after octreotide discontinued.
Kim-Sing et al. (1994)[16]	Descriptive	1	AIDS patient with severe, watery diarrhea received octreotide 500 mcg SC every 8 hours for 4 days, then dose tapered 300 mcg/day every 4 days to find minimally effective dose. Patient previously given antidiarrheals and specific antimycobacterial therapy without response.	Daily of bowel movements decreased from 10-15 to < 5 and daily stool volume went from 4.25 L to 2.3 L during therapy with octreotide 500 mcg SC Q 8 hours. Patient became continent and ambulatory. When dose reduced < 200 mcg SC Q 8 hours, bowel movements increased to 6-8/day.	V	None.
Kreinik et al. (1991)[22]	Descriptive	1	AIDS patient with cryptosporidial diarrhea refractory to opiate antidiarrheals given octreotide 100 mcg SC TID 300 mcg SC TID, and 150-400 mcg daily by IV infusion.	Stool frequency was 10-12/day with volumes 1 L/stool. No response with octreotide 100 mcg SC TID; patient did not tolerate 300 mcg SC dose. Octreotide 150 mcg/day by IV infusion decreased stool frequency to 4/day for 3 weeks then dosage increase to 300 mcg/day required. After 1 week, dosage increase to 400 mcg/day required to maintain stool frequency at 3-4/day.	V	Diarrhea recurred when octreotide stopped for brief period. Drug restarted and patient maintained on IV octreotide for 5 months.
Rene et al. (1986)[21]	Descriptive	4	AIDS patients with cryptosporidial diarrhea given octreotide 100 mcg SC BID for 3-7 days.	Daily stool output decreased significantly in 2/4 patients and did not rebound upon discontinuation. Other two patients had no change in stool volume.	IV	Two patients who did not respond were also infected with colonic *Cytomegalovirus*.
Robinson et al. (1988)[19]	Descriptive	1	AIDS patient with diarrhea given octreotide 50 mcg SC BID. Dose titrated up to 200 mcg SC TID as needed and continued 10 weeks.	Stool frequency decreased from 8-10 liquid stools/day at baseline to 3 semi-formed stools/day on octreotide (dose not specified).	V	Diarrhea recurred when dose reduced to 100 mcg/day.

TABLE 1 (continued)

Reference	Study Design	n	Intervention	Results	Level of Evidence	Comments
Romeu et al. (1991)[20]	Prospective, open-label, dose-finding	29	AIDS patients with diarrhea after a week of antidiarrheals given octreotide 50 mcg SC TID. If no or partial response, dose increased Q 48 hours to 100, 250, or 500 mcg SC TID. Once controlled, dose continued 4 weeks. Complete response defined as 2 bowel movements daily with increased consistency; partial response if 50% reduction in bowel movements or increased stool consistency. Diarrhea defined as 3 unformed bowel movements daily. Duration of diarrhea was 0.5-28.0 months.	Response occurred in 19/25 (76%) evaluable patients: complete response in 10 patients and partial response in 9 patients. No responses with octreotide 50 mcg SC TID: median dose for response was 100 mcg SC TID. Partial responders tended to require higher doses than complete responders. Daily number of stools was 8.8 ± 5.0 at baseline. Patients treated a mean of 4.2 ± 4.2 months (range, 1-16) with a mean response duration of 4.4 ± 4.5 months.	IV	72% (13/18) of patients with enteric cryptosporidium infection responded: complete response in 22% (4/18), partial response in 50% (9/18). Compared with this group, more patients with non-cryptosporidial enteritis had complete rather than partial response (p = 0.007).
Vinik et al. (1986)[15]	Descriptive	2	Male patients with carcinoid syndrome received octreotide doses ranging from 50 mcg SC BID to 150 mcg SC every 8 hours for 5-8 months.	No response to 50 mcg SQ BID in 1 patient. Symptoms resolved at 150 mcg SQ BID. Symptoms reduced in the other patient with 50 mcg SQ Q8H; dose increased to 150 mcg SQ Q8H for inadequate tumor response.	V	None.
		1	Female patient with VIPoma received octreotide 200 mcg SC QID for 2 months then 100 mcg SC QID for at least 2 months.	Bowel movements decreased to 1-2 formed stools daily. Daily stool volume decreased from 9 L of watery diarrhea to 0.5 L.	V	None.

Abbreviations: AIDS = acquired immunodefiency syndrome; BID = twice daily; IV = intravenously administered; PO = orally administered; QID = four times daily; SC = subcutaneously administered; TID = three times daily; VIPoma = vasoactive intestinal peptide tumor

Key to Level of Evidence classification:
Level I   Randomized trials with low false-positive (alpha) and low false-negative (beta errors); high power
Level II   Randomized trials with high false-positive (alpha) and/or high false-negative (beta errors); low power
Level III   Nonrandomized concurrent cohort comparisons between contemporaneous patients who did and did not receive a given intervention
Level IV   Nonrandomized historical cohort comparisons between current patients who did receive the intervention and patients (from the same institution or from the literature) who did not
Level V   Case series without control subjects

TABLE 2 Drug Therapy for Managing Diarrhea in Palliative Care[1-3,8,9,27,28]

Drug	Pharmacologic Effect	Indication	Dosing Regimen	AWP per Day of Therapy[#]
aspirin 325 mg tablets	Prostaglandin inhibitor	Radiation-induced diarrhea	325 mg po every 4-6 hours (Enteric-coated 325 mg tablets also available)	$0.06-0.09 $0.08-0.12
bismuth subsalicylate (PeptoBismol) 262 mg caplets, 262 mg chewable tablets	Prostaglandin inhibitor; antibacterial	Symptom control	524 mg po every 30-60 minutes, up to 5000 mg/day (Liquid product available: 262 mg/15 ml liquid and 524 mg/15 ml liquid)	$0.18-1.74 $0.25-2.38 $0.15-1.42
cholestyramine powder[††] (Questran, Prevalite)	Bile acid sequestrant	Diarrhea due to ileal resection or radiation	4-12 g po tid	$2.53-7.58 (powder)[†] $3.50-10.50 (packets)
codeine sulfate 15 mg, 30 mg, 60 m tablets	Opioid agonist	Symptom control	15-60 mg PO every 4-6 hours	$1.36-5.42
cyproheptadine 4 mg tablets (Periactin)	Peripheral serotonin antagonist	Carcinoid syndrome	4 mg PO tid-qid (syrup: 2 mg/5 mL)	$0.19-0.25 $0.62-0.82
diphenoxylate/atropine 2.5/0.025 mg tablet (Lomotil)	Opioid agonist anticholinergic combination	Symptom control	2.5-5.0 mg diphenoxylate q 4-6 h (Liquid: 2.5 mg diphenoxylate, 0.025 mg atropine/5 mL liquid)	$0.29-0.88 $4.68-14.03
hydrocortisone 100 mg/60 mL retention enema	Corticosteroid	Radiation colitis, tumor invasion	100 mg PR nightly	$9.16
kaolin/pectin suspension	Adsorbent/absorbent combination	Symptom control	30-60 mL PO every 4 hours	$1.87-3.74
Kaolin, pectin and attapuluigite suspension (Kaopectate)	Adsorbent/absorbent combination	Symptom control	30-60 mL PO every 4 hours	$2.86-5.72
lipase 4,500 units/protease 25,000 units/amylase 20,000 units (Pancrease)	Pancreatic enzyme replacement	Fat malabsorption, steatorrhea	1-3 capsules PO with meals, 1 capsule with snacks; titrate prn	$1.77-3.90 (Assuming 3 meals and 2 snacks/day)

TABLE 2 (continued)

Drug	Pharmacologic Effect	Indication	Dosing Regimen	AWP per Day of Therapy[#]
loperamide 2 mg tablets, capsules (Imodium)	Opioid agonist	Symptom control	4 mg PO, then 2-4 mg PO q 4-6 h Liquid: 1 mg per 5 mL	$2.89-6.92 $2.08-4.98
mesalamine 250 mg capsules (Pentasa), 400 mg tablets (Asacol)	Prostaglandin inhibitor	Ulcerative colitis	4 cr capsules PO qid 1-2 dr tablets PO tid	$5.88 $1.85-3.71
methylcellulose 2g/15 mL powder (Citrucel)[†]	Bulk-forming agent	Symptom control	1 tablespoon PO q day-tid	$0.06-0.20 (powder) $0.38-1.14 (packets)
octreotide (Sandostatin)	Somatostatin analog	Carcinoid tumors, vipomas, aids-related diarrhea	Aids: 50-500 mcg SC tid (starting dose 50-100 mcg SC bid) Carcinoid: 100-600 mcg SC in 2-4 divided doses Vipoma: 200-300 mcg SC in 2-4 divided doses	AIDS: $15.39-151.51 Carcinoid: $10.26-60.60 (mdv) $10.42-76.30 (sdv) Vipoma: $20.52-30.78 (mdv) $19.07-38.15 (sdv)
Opium tincture, deodorized 10%	Opioid agonist	Symptom control	0.6-1.2 ml PO every 4-6 hours	$0.99-2.96
psyllium mucilloid, 3.4 g (Metamucil)	Bulk-forming agent	Symptom control	3.4 g psyllium PO BID-TID	$0.10-0.15 (powder) $0.13-0.19 (SF powder) $0.51-0.76 (packets)

Abbreviations: AIDS = acquired immunodeficiency syndrome; BID = twice daily; CR = controlled release; DR = delayed release; MDV = multiple-dose vial; PO = orally administered; PR = rectally administered; QD = once daily; QID = four times daily; SC = subcutaneously administered; SDV = single-dose vial; SF = sugar-free; TID = three times daily; VIPoma = vasoactive intestinal peptide tumor

[†] Regular and sugar-free products available. Average wholesale price the same for both.
[‡] Dosing based on cholestyramine content of powder.

Questran and generic product contain 4 g anhydrous cholestyramine resin per 9 g powder
Questran Light and sugar-free generic product contains 4 g anhydrous cholestyramine resin per 5 g powder.

[#] Average Wholesale Price, 1999 (cost to pharmacy)

REFERENCES

1. Driscoll CE. Symptom control in terminal illness. Primary Care. 1987;14:353-63.

2. Levy MH, Catalano RB. Control of common physical symptoms other than pain in patients with terminal disease. Seminars in Oncology. 1985;12:411-30.

3. Rousseau P. Nonpain symptom management in terminal care. Clin Geriatr Med. 1996;12:313-27.

4. Sykes NP. Constipation and diarrhoea. In: Doyle D, Hanks GWC, MacDonald N, eds. Oxford Textbook of Palliative Medicine. New York, NY: Oxford University Press; 1993:299-310.

5. Connolly G, Shanson D, Hawkins D, Harcourt-Webster J, Gazzard B. Non-cryptosporidial diarrhoea in human immunodeficiency virus (HIV) infected patients. Gut. 1989;30:195-200.

6. Holmes S. Use of a modified symptom distress scale in assessment of the cancer patient. Int J Nurs Stud. 1989;26:69-79.

7. Anderson DM. Dorland's Illustrated Medical Dictionary. 28th ed. ed. Philadelphia, PA: W.B. Saunders Company; 1994.

8. McGowan I, Allason-Jones E. Symptomatic management of HIV associated gastrointestinal disease. Cancer Surv. 1994;21:157-77.

9. Threlkeld D, Hageman R, Brantley A, et al. Drug Facts and Comparisons. St. Louis: Facts and Comparisons; 1997.

10. Fine K. Pathophysiology/Diagnosis/Management. In: Feldman M, Sleisenger M, Scharschmidt B, eds. Sleisenger and Fordtran's Gastrointestinal and Liver Disease. Philadelphia, PA: W. B. Saunders Company; 1998.

11. Condon J, Wolverson R, South M, Brinkley D. Radiation diarrhoea and cholestyramine. Postgrad Med J. 1978;54:838-9.

12. Mennie A, Dalley V, Dinneen L, Collier H. Treatment of radiation-induced gastrointestinal distress with acetylsalicylate. Lancet 1975. 1975;2:942-3.

13. Geelhoed G, Bass B, Mertz S, Becker K. Somatostatin analog: effects on hypergastrinemia and hypercalcitoninemia. Surgery. 1986;100:962-70.

14. Brabant G, Muller M, Rotsch M, Havemann K, Schmidt F, Hesch R. Treatment of carcinoid syndrome and VIPoma with a long-acting somatorstatin analogue (SMS 201-995). Scand J Gastroenterol. 1986;21:177-80.

15. Vinik A, Tsai S, Moattari A, Cheung P, Eckhauser F, Cho K. Somatostatin analogue (SMS 201-995) in the management of gastroenteropancreatic tumors and diarrhea syndromes. Am J Med. 1986;81:23-40.

16. Kim-Sing A, Yoshida E, Whittaker J. Palliative high-dose octreotide in a case of severe AIDS-related diarrhea. Ann Pharmacother. 1994;28:806-7.

17. Fanning M, Monte M, Sutherland L, Broadhead M, Murphy G, Harris A. Pilot study of Sandostatin (octreotide) therapy of refractory HIV-associated diarrhea. Dig Dis Sci. 1991;36:476-80.

18. Cello J, Grendell J, Basuk P. Effect of octreotide on refractory AIDS-associated diarrhea. A prospective, multicenter clinical trial. Ann Int Med. 1991;115:705-10.

19. Robinson E, Fogel R. SMS 201-995, a somatostatin analogue, and diarrhoea in the acquired immunodeficiency syndrome. Ann Intern Med. 1988;109:680-1.

20. Romeu J, Miro J, Cirera G. Efficacy of octreotide in the management of chronic diarrhoea in AIDS. AIDS. 1991;5:1495-9.

21. Rene E, Regnier B, Laine M, Bonfils S. Somatostatin and cryptosporidial diarrhoea during AIDS. Can J Physiol Pharmacol. 1986;64 (suppl):70.

22. Kreinik G, Burstein O, Landor M, Bernstein L, Weiss L, Wittner M. Successful management of intractable cryptosporidial diarrhoea with intravenous octreotide, a somatostatin analogue. AIDS. 1991;5:765-7.

23. Katz M, Erstad B, Rose C. Treatment of severe cryptosporidium-related diarrhea with octreotide in a patient with AIDS. Drug Intell Clin Pharm. 1988;22:134-6.

24. Cook D, Kelton J, Stanisz A, Collins S. Somatostatin treatment for cryptosporidial diarrhoea in a patient with the acquired immunodeficiency syndrome (AIDS). Ann Intern Med. 1988;108:708-9.

25. Clotet B, Cofan F, Materola J, Foz M. Efficacy of the somatostatin analogue (SMS-201-995), Sandostatin, for cryptosporidial diarrhoea in patients with AIDS. AIDS. 1989;3:857-8.

26. Brunton L. Agents affecting gastrointestinal water flux and motility; emesis an antiemetics; bile acids and pancreatic enzymes. In: Hardman J, Limbird L, Molinoff P, Ruddon R, Gilman A, eds. Goodman & Gilman's The Pharmacological Basis of Therapeutics. 9th edition, New York: McGraw-Hill; 1996:901-36.

27. Mercadante S. The role of octreotide in palliative care. J Pain Symptom Manage. 1994;9:406-11.

Dyspnea in Palliative Care Patients

Linda S. Tyler

SUMMARY. Dyspnea is perhaps the most distressing symptom experienced by palliative care patients. Potential underlying causes are listed. Supportive therapy is important. Oxygen and opioids are the most common therapies for dyspnea, but several other drugs and drug classes have been used to help manage the symptom. Evaluation instruments that have been used for the symptom are described. Some open research questions are listed. A treatment algorithm, evidence tables and drug therapy tables which include drug costs are presented. *[Article copies available for a fee from The Haworth Document Delivery Service: 1-800-342-9678. E-mail address: getinfo@haworthpressinc.com <Website: http://www.haworthpressinc.com>]*

KEYWORDS. Dyspnea, breathing, air hunger, palliative care, terminal care, dying, supportive care, drug therapy, non-pharmacological therapy, etiology, evidence, costs, algorithm, oxygen, opioids, morphine, continuous infusion, nebulized, benzodiazepines, diazepam, anticholinergic agents, atropine, hyoscyamine, corticosteroids, steroids, prednisone, dexamethasone, phenothiazines, chlorpromazine, promethazine, local anesthetics, lidocaine, diuretics, furosemide, bronchodilators, albuterol, iproatropium, aminophylline, theophylline, systematic review

Linda S. Tyler, PharmD, is Professor, College of Pharmacy; and Manager, Drug Information Service, Department of Pharmacy Services, University Hospitals and Clinics; University of Utah Health Sciences Center, Salt Lake City, UT.

Address correspondence to: Arthur G. Lipman, PharmD, College of Pharmacy and Pain Management Center, 30 S 2000 E RM 258, University of Utah Health Sciences Center, Salt Lake City, UT 84112-5820 (E-mail: alipman@pharm.utah.edu).

[Haworth co-indexing entry note]: "Dyspnea in Palliative Care Patients." Tyler, Linda S. Co-published simultaneously in *Journal of Pharmaceutical Care in Pain & Symptom Control* (Pharmaceutical Products Press, an imprint of The Haworth Press, Inc.) Vol. 7, No. 4, 1999, pp. 109-127; and: *Evidence Based Symptom Control in Palliative Care: Systematic Reviews and Validated Clinical Practice Guidelines for 15 Common Problems in Patients with Life Limiting Disease* (ed: Arthur G. Lipman, Kenneth C. Jackson II, and Linda S. Tyler) Pharmaceutical Products Press, an imprint of The Haworth Press, Inc., 2000, pp. 109-127. Single or multiple copies of this article are available for a fee from The Haworth Document Delivery Service [1-800-342-9678, 9:00 a.m. 5:00 p.m. (EST). E-mail address: getinfo@haworthpressinc.com].

Algorithm for Managing Dyspea

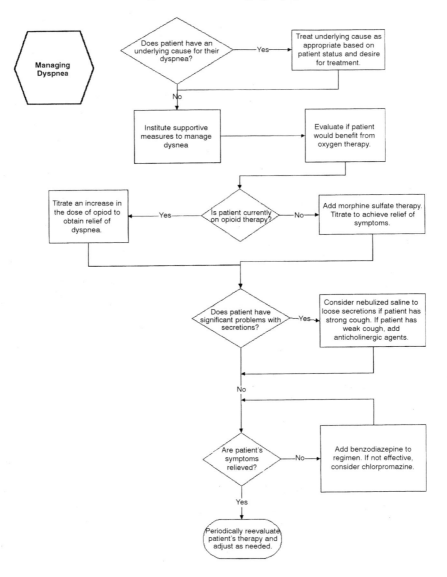

Dyspnea is reported to occur in 30-70%[2,3] of patients dying of cancer. The pathophysiology of dyspnea in palliative care is complex.[1,2] When present, it is rated as moderate to severe (clinically important for the patient) 63% of the time.[4] It is more common in patients with lung, colorectal, and breast cancer.[3,5] In one study, patients with dyspnea had lung or pleural involvement 39% of the time.[3]

Several authors[5,6] have suggested that for many patients the onset of dyspnea may represent the patient's moving to the terminal phase of their disease. Escalante[5] evaluated 122 patients who presented to the emergency room of a major cancer center with dyspnea as the presenting symptom. Of these patients, 68% had uncontrolled progressive disease, and 50% had more than one etiology for their dyspnea. Thirty-two percent of these patients died on the initial hospitalization. The overall median survival was 12 weeks. In lung cancer patients with dyspnea, 31% died within two weeks; the medial survival was 4 weeks. Higginson[6] summarized the symptoms of 86 patients referred to a terminal care support team. Twenty-one percent of patients developed dyspnea as they approached death and dyspnea was described as their most severe symptom. While the pain symptom scores of the patients decreased, those of dyspnea did not. Of the 13 patients with dyspnea as their major symptom at referral, 6 died within 2 weeks of referral. Lynn[7] interviewed the family members of 3,357 patients who were older or seriously ill concerning the death experience. More than half of the patients had severe dyspnea in the last 3 days of life. Fatigue and dyspnea were the most commonly reported symptoms.

Many treatment strategies have been suggested for managing dyspnea, but few data are available that evaluate these therapies in palliative care. Table 1 summaries the available evidence.

EVALUATE THE CAUSES OF DYSPNEA
AND TREAT THE UNDERLYING CAUSE WHEN POSSIBLE

Each patient with dyspnea should be evaluated for causes as well as other factors that may be contributing the dyspnea. Anxiety is frequently increased in patients with dyspnea; likewise, patients with anxiety may have dyspnea. Pain, fatigue, anxiety, depression, loss of appetite, and sleep disorders are often concomitant symptoms. Cough or hiccups may accompany the dyspnea.

The following considerations should be assessed when attempting

TABLE 1. Drug Therapy for Managing Dyspnea in Palliative Care–Evidence Tables

Reference	Study Design	n	Intervention	Results	Level of Evidence	Comments
Oxygen						
Bruera (1993)[12]	Experimental: Cross-over, double-blind	14	Terminally ill cancer patients with dyspnea, capable of participating in a study, were randomized to receive either oxygen or air via mask. Patients were evaluated 5 minutes after achieving stable oxygen saturation. Patients then received the alternate therapy. Patients were randomized a second time. Each patient had 4 total evaluation periods, two with each therapy. Patients were evaluated using a dyspnea VAS scale (0-100) and global rating score.	The mean VAS scores showed improvement in dyspnea symptoms by 11 from baseline to oxygen, and 20 from air to oxygen (15.9 in the second phase) (p values <0.001). Twelve patients preferred oxygen. Patients reported little to no benefit when receiving air, and moderate to much benefit during oxygen on the global rating score.	II	small sample size
Bruera (1990)[20]	Descriptive	20	Patients with dyspnea dying from lung cancer were candidates for the study. Prior to the next dose of opioids for pain (15 patients) or when they entered the study (5 patients), they were evaluated (dyspnea VAS 0-100), pulse oximetry, respiratory effort, and pain. For patients already receiving opioids, 2.5 times the equivalent dose was administered as morphine. For the other patients, 5 mg was administered.	Dyspnea score improved by a mean of 34 (p < 0.001). No difference in patients receiving opioids and those not were noted. No deterioration in oxygen saturation, pCO_2, respiratory rate or effort were noted.	V	
Bruera (1993)[29]	Experimental: cross-over, double blind	10	Terminal cancer patients with dyspnea were randomized to receive morphine or placebo. The next day they received the alternate treatment. All were receiving morphine for pain. The morphine dose was calculated to be 50% greater than their usual dose. Dyspnea was evaluated using VAS scores from 0-100.	Dyspnea symptoms improved by 11 points at 30 minutes, 16 at 45 minutes and 14 at one hour (all p values <0.02 compared to baseline). No change in respiratory rate or oxygen saturation was noted. Morphine was chosen as more effective by 9 patients and 8 physicians.	II	
Morphine continuous infusion						
Cohen, (1991)[18]	Descriptive	8	Patients had sever dyspnea unrelieved by non-opioids and intermittent bolus opioids. Morphine 1-2 mg was administered every 5-10 minutes until relief of symptoms. Continuous infusion morphine was initiated based on initial doses used. Dose was titrated to relieve symptoms.	Dyspnea relief was "good" in 6 patients, moderate in one, and poor in one. Five were somnolent on the doses needed to relieve dyspnea symptoms. ABG's worsened in most patients.	V	

Morphine and Chlorpromazine

Ventafridda, (1990)[26]	Descriptive	5	Patients with advanced cancer disease without pain who had dyspnea were treated with morphine hydrochloride 10 mg IM and chlorpromazine 25 mg (route not specified).	Patients demonstrated "satisfactory" results. While VAS scores are reported as being measured, the data are not presented.	V

Morphine—nebulized

Francombe (1993)[22]	Descriptive	4	Initial dose was morphine 2.5 mg (2 patients with end stage heart failure) or 5 mg (2 with end stage lung disease) in 2 mL sterile water administered c 4 h to relieve severe dyspnea. Dose was increased to 25 mg and 17.5 mg over two weeks to maintain control in the lung disease patients; and used intermittently to treat heart failure patients.	Three patients had good control of their symptoms and continued on therapy until their death. One patient in heart failure initially responded, but reported a smothering feeling as her condition deteriorated and was switched to subcutaneous injections.	V
Francombe (1994)[23]	Descriptive	3	Three terminally ill cancer patients received nebulized opioids; one received morphine 5 mg, one hydromorphone 8 mg, and one aneridine 25 mg. All were administered with 2 mL of sterile water.	Patients responded well to therapy.	V
Francombe (1994)[24]	Descriptive	54	Reviewed the charts of 54 terminally ill patients who received nebulized opioids for relief of dyspnea.	34 patients received morphine, 17 hydromorphone, 2 codeine and 1 anileridine. Patients received the same opioid they got for pain relief or morphine if they were not on opioids. 34 patients had subjective improvement noted in their charts, 12 received 1 or 2 doses then discontinued therapy, 8 had conflicting information in chart concerning clinical response	V

Key to Level of Evidence classification:

Level I   Randomized trials with low false-positive (alpha) and low false-negative (beta errors); high power

Level II   Randomized trials with high false-positive (alpha) and/or high false-negative (beta errors); low power

Level III   Nonrandomized concurrent cohort comparisons between contemporaneous patients who did and did not receive a given intervert on

Level IV   Nonrandomized historical cohort comparisons between current patients who did receive the intervention and patients (from the same institution or from the literature) who did not

Level V   Case series without control subjects

to identify the underlying causes that may cause dyspnea.[2,8,9] Whether or not to treat these causes is a decision that must be made in conjunction with the patient, their family, and their care providers.

- Infection
- Consider if patient presents with fever, chills, or purulent sputum. Treat with appropriate antibiotics, antipyretics, and other supportive care as indicated.
- Pleural effusion
- Consider if the patient also presents with breath sounds changing by location or deviated trachea. Depending on the patient's status, thoracentesis or sclero-therapy may be helpful.
- Obstruction
- Consider if the patient has progressive or rapidly increasing dyspnea, noisy breathing, chronic cough. Corticosteroids may beneficial in these patients. Many patients may benefit from palliative radiotherapy or chemotherapy. Students have been used in some patients to maintain the patency of the airway.
- Volume overload
- Consider if patient has rales and other signs of fluid overload. Diuretics are helpful in many patients. Fluid restriction may be indicated as well.
- Thick secretions
- If the patient has a strong cough reflex, nebulized saline may be useful to loosen secretions. Anticholinergic agents may be useful to dry secretions.
- Anemia
- Consider if patient has a low hemoglobin, or presents with general fatigue, weakness, headache, or rapid heart rate. Transfusions would be used if treatment is desired.
- Pulmonary emboli
- Consider if patient has sudden onset of symptoms with rapid breathing, rapid heart rate, cough, chest pain, or blood in sputum.
- Pericardial effusion
- Consider if patient has chest pain relieved by leaning forward, weakness, pleural effusion, edema, or distension of neck vein. Pericardial centesis may be useful in some patients
- Ascites

- Consider if dyspnea is accompanied by abdominal distension and tenderness. Fluid restriction should be considered for these patients.
- Superior vena cava syndrome
- Consider if distended neck veins, facial or arm swelling, cough, noisy breathing, decreased consciousness. Onset can be rapid and may constitute an oncologic emergency. High dose corticosteroids may be effective in reducing the edema. Radiation therapy may also be indicated.
- Lymphangitis carcinomatosis

The onset may be insidious or viewed as progression of the disease. Chest X-rays are usually consistent with pulmonary congestion without an enlarged heart. Radiation therapy may be useful. High dose corticosteroids have been used, but may worsen symptoms by causing fluid retention. The symptomatic treatment as outlined below may be the best therapy. It is useful to consider drug or other therapy as a potential cause of dyspnea. Radiotherapy and chemotherapy may induce pulmonary toxicity.[10] Management is usually symptomatic.

IMPLEMENT SUPPORTIVE THERAPY

The following non-pharmacologic therapies have been recommended as being beneficial in the management of dyspnea.[8,9] Some may not be appropriate based on the patient's individual circumstances or preferences.

- Find the position that makes the patient the most comfortable. For many patients, keeping head and torso elevated helps. If the patient just has one lung involved, lying on one side or the other may be more comfortable (usually with the affected lung down).
- Limit activity and reduce the need for exertion. Space activities apart. Prioritize activities. Usual care activities may need to be spread out. Arrange for readily available help.
- Improve air circulation. Create a draft (i.e., use a table fan, open windows).
- Use a humidifier.
- A cooler room temperature may be preferable.
- Eliminate respiratory irritants such as smoking.

- Evaluate and manage anxiety.
- Help the patient and family member understand dyspnea and the treatment strategies available. Identify trigger factors if possible.
- Use breathing re-training, relaxation, coping, and adaptation strategies. Corner et al.[11] found that these strategies significantly improved symptoms compared to a control group in lung cancer patients.

TREAT DYSPNEA PHARMACOLOGICALLY

Numerous pharmacologic modalities have been recommended in the management of dyspnea. These are summarized in Table 2 and are discussed below.

Oxygen

Oxygen therapy may be useful in many patients. Its role, however, is controversial. It is indicated in patients with hypoxemia, but diagnosing and monitoring for this require special considerations. Drawing arterial blood gases may be painful for patients. Determining oxygen saturation using a pulse oximeter is preferable in palliative care because it is non-invasive.

Oxygen may not be needed in many patients because other therapy (opioids) is very effective.[9] If oxygen is administered, a nasal cannula is preferred. Masks make some patients feel isolated and frightened. Oxygen may also have a placebo effect. In some patient care settings, it may be expensive and cumbersome.

Bruera[12] studied the effects of oxygen compared to air in 14 patients with cancer dyspnea in a randomized double-blind cross-over trial (Table 1). All patients had received oxygen via nasal cannula prior to the study. Patients were randomized to treatment, crossed over to the other treatment, then randomized a second time receive a second set of each treatment. The mean VAS scores (scale 0-100) showed improvement in dyspnea symptoms by 11 from baseline to oxygen, and 20 from air to oxygen (15.9 in the second phase) (p values < 0.001). Twelve patients preferred oxygen. Patients reported little to no benefit when receiving air, and moderate to great benefit on the global rating scale when receiving oxygen. Based on this study, others[13,14]

TABLE 2. Drug Therapy for Managing Dyspnea in Palliative Care

Drug Therapy	Indications for Use	Dosing Regimen	AWP per Day of Therapy#
oxygen	Patients with hypoxia Use in other patients controversial	Initial dose: 4 L/min via nasal cannula	
Opioids morphine	Mainstay of therapy in patients who do not have an underlying cause of dyspnea which can be treated.	Doses titrated based on effect. Initial dosing recommendations for patients not already taking opioids. (See text if currently taking opioids)	
Benzodiazepines diazepam (Valium)	Unclear if have a mechanism for relieving dyspnea besides their anxiolytic activity. Use as an adjunctive to morphine therapy, especially in patients with anxiety.	Effects are titrated to patient effect. 2-5 mg PO hs 2 mg po q12h 2 mg IV q12	$0.02 $0.04 $5.88
Anticholinergic agents hyoscyamine atropine	Use to decrease secretions. Especially useful in patients with weak cough.	0.125 mg PO or SL q8h 0.4-1 mg IV, IM or SQ q4-8h	$0.36 $1.46-2.93
Corticosteroids Prednisone Dexamethasone (Decadron)	Use in patients with bronchospasm, edema, lymphangitis carcinomatosa, laryngeal stricture, tracheal or bronchial obstruction or superior vena cava syndrome	20-40 mg/d PO 20 mg PO initially, 8 mg PO bid (morning and noon)	$0.14-0.28 20 mg = $1.10 8 mg bid = $0.88 $0.44 $0.45-0.90
Phenothiazines chlorpromazine (Thorazine) promethazine (Phenergan)	Recommended for patients who do not respond to any of the above therapies.	12.5 mg IV q4-12 h or 25 mg PR q4-12h 25 mg PO q4-6h 25 mg IV q4-6h 25-50 mg PR q4-6h	$1.05-3.14 $11.80-17.70 $0.10-0.15 $2.04-3.06 $8.83-15.61
Local anesthetics (nebulized) lidocaine (Xylocaine)	occasionally recommend in patients who do not respond to any of the above therapies	4 mL of 10% solution (400 mg)	$3.46

TABLE 2 (continued)

Drug Therapy	Indications for Use	Dosing Regimen	AWP per Day of Therapy#
Diuretics furosemide (Lasix)	For patients with congestive heart failure or fluid overload.	20-80 mg IV	$2.03-4.12
Bronchodilators (representative drugs listed) albuterol (Proventil, Ventolin)	Use in patients with evidence of bronchospasm or chronic obstructive pulmonary disease.	2-4 puffs q 4-6 h 2.5 mg q 6-8h	$0.86-2.66 {$22.20/17 G inhaler (200 puffs)} $3.60-4.80
ipratropium bromide (Atrovent)		2 puffs q6h 250-500 mcg q6-8h	$1.16 ($29.12/inhaler 200 puffs) $5.88-7.81
aminophylline		(Representative doses for a 70 kg patient given; please check specific dosing guidelines for a patient. acute bronchospasm: 6 mg/kg loading dose; 0.6 mg/kg/hr IV for First 12 hours then 0.3 mg/kg/hr	$10.78 for first 24 hours
theophylline		chronic dosing: 13 mg/kg/d	$1.35

Average Wholesale Price, 1999 (cost to pharmacy)

118

have recommended that oxygen may improve patients' symptoms. However, this study was conducted for a short time interval. Some recommend it as part of their standard approach to patients.[15]

Opioids

Opioid therapy is the main therapy recommended in managing dyspnea. Several mechanisms of action may be responsible for the effect. Opioids decrease the perception of breathlessness. They also decrease the ventilatory drive by decreasing the responsiveness to hypercapnia and hypoxia, and decrease oxygen consumption. Morphine has vasodilation activity which is known to benefit patients in heart failure, but it is not known if this effect is beneficial in dyspnea from other causes.[2] Table 1 summarizes the studies that have been conducted evaluating morphine. These are all descriptive reports in small numbers of patients.

Since many patients are already receiving opioid therapy for pain, several strategies for using these drugs are indicated based on existing therapy and severity of dyspnea. Likewise, many patients may have intermittent symptoms, especially related to activity. For patients with intermittent symptoms, as needed regimens may be the best approach. However, regular dosing should be used for those patients with persistent symptoms.

In patients with mild dyspnea who are taking no opioids, dyspnea may be managed by taking an oral opioid such as morphine 5 mg q4h with an additional dose of 5 mg every 2 hours prn.[9] Acetaminophen 325 mg with codeine 30 mg 1 tablet every 4 hours has been used with an additional dose of 30 mg every 2 hours prn. Some authors report that codeine is not effective for dyspnea.[2]

In patients with severe dyspnea, or dyspnea being treated with "weak" opioids, e.g., propoxyphene, codeine, changing to a strong opioid such as morphine may provide relief. Potential regimens include oxycodone 3-10 mg every 4 hours and prn; morphine syrup 3-10 mg q 4 hours and prn; and hydromorphone 0.5-2 mg q4h prn.[9] Other authors recommend morphine sulfate 5 mg po every 4 hours. The dose can be increased by 5 mg every day until symptoms are relieved.[16] Walsh[17] recommends starting morphine sulfate sustained release 15 mg every 12 hours. If oral opioids are not tolerated, subcutaneous therapy can be used.

Continuous infusion therapy also been used. Boluses of morphine sulfate 1 to 2 mg every 5 to 10 minutes may be administered until the dyspnea is relieved. In one report, the total cumulative dose necessary to control the dyspnea was calculated and one-half of that dose per hour was administered as a continuous infusion.[18] Patients with exacerbations received a 25% increase in their dose. If excessive somnolence occurred or the respiratory rate was less than 10 breaths per minute, the dose was decreased by 50%. If patients developed tolerance, the dose was increased 25% after 1 to 2 days. For patients with severe dyspnea who were being treated with strong opioids, a suggested dosing adjustment is to increase the dose by 50% every 4 to 12 hours until the patient experiences relief.[9]

It is not clear if opioids decrease respiratory function in relieving the symptoms of dyspnea. Several authors[17,19] cite Bruera et al.[20] as evidence that morphine does not cause a decrease in respiratory parameters when used to treat dyspnea. However, the cited study only used a single dose of morphine sulfate 5 mg in patients not receiving opioids and 2.5 times the usual opioid dose in patients taking opioids. Cohen et al.[18] studied patients over a longer time period and found that respiratory function decreased in patients, but justified the therapy as important in relieving symptoms. Respiratory depression need not be problematic if the amount of morphine is titrated to patient response rather than using predetermined doses.[21]

Farncombe published several reports on the use of nebulized opioids for managing dyspnea.[22-24] This is an alternative route of administration for patients who cannot take oral medications or IV. Many patients demonstrated improvement of their symptoms (Table 1). Initial doses used were morphine sulfate 5 mg in 2 mL sterile water (n = 34). If patients were receiving opioids for pain, those drugs were used if possible (hydromorphine 1 mg, n = 17; codeine 15 mg, n = 2). Only one patient responded to codeine. Fentanyl has also been used (50-100 mcg via nebulization).[2] Some patients may prefer a nebulized route of administration. This route has a onset of action within 2-5 minutes.[2] Nebulization also may cause a local effect, but this has not been proven. It is unclear if patients may become less sedated with this route of administration.[2] Because morphine may cause bronchospasm, the first dose should probably be administered in a setting where bronchospasm can be managed.

While morphine is the drug most commonly described in the literature, other opioids may be used, especially if the patient is already stabilized on another opioid for pain control. Some authors suggest fentanyl, especially if the patient is experiencing histamine release with morphine sulfate.[21,25] Fentanyl has also been used by an inhalation route of administration.

Naloxone should be used extremely cautiously in terminally ill patients.[9,16] Naloxone use is recommended in cases of accidental overdose and should not be used to completely reverse the opioid effects. Naloxone can precipitate return of extreme pain and dyspnea, as well as withdrawal effects. Storey[9] recommends using a dilution of naloxone of 0.4 mg/mL naloxone diluted to 10 mL with saline; administer 1 mL every 5 minutes until partial reversal is observed. It may be necessary to repeat this dose since naloxone has a short half-life.

Benzodiazepines

Many authors recommend benzodiazepines as the next class of drugs to consider in patients with dyspnea. Since anxiety commonly accompanies dyspnea, the rational for these drugs is to decrease anxiety. Other authors[2,13] suggest that there may be additional, unidentified mechanisms which help to explain the effectiveness of benzodiazepines in relieving dyspnea. No studies have been done specifically in dyspnea in the terminally ill patient. Walsh[17] recommends diazepam because its long half-life is convenient, permitting administration of 2 mg every 12 hours. Daily diazepam doses of 2 and 5 mg at bedtime may also relieve symptoms.[13]

Lorazepam has a shorter half-life which may make it easier to use in some patients.[2,9] While it may be administered orally, it may also be administered sublingually and parenterally. Campbell[14] recommended lorazepam as a 2 to 4 mg bolus with a 1 to 3 mg per hour constant infusion. Storey also recommended midazolam beginning with a dose of 0.25 mg per hour subcutaneously and rapidly increased to the desired effect. Two to 3 mg per hour may be necessary.[9] Midazolam as a 2 to 4 mg bolus followed by 2 to 5 mg per hour titrated to patient response is another recommended regimen.[14] Midazolam has an amnesic effect which may be useful in some patients.

Anticholinergic Agents

In patients with secretions, the following therapies may be beneficial. If the cough reflex is strong, secretions may be loosened with nebulized saline. If the cough is weak, the secretions may be dried by use of an anticholinergic agent. Some authors suggest hyoscyamine 0.125 mg orally or sublingually every 8 hours, transdermal scopolamine 1 to 3 patches every 3 days, or add glycopyrrolate 0.4 to1.0 mg per day to an existing subcutaneous infusions, or 0.2 mg q 3 hours SC or IV every 3 hours.[9] Atropine 0.4 to1 mg q 4 to 8h may also be used.[16]

Corticosteroids

Glucocorticosteroids are recommended in patients who may have bronchospasm, edema, lymphangitis carcinomatosa, laryngeal stricture, tracheal or bronchial obstruction, or superior vena cava syndrome. Prednisone 20 to 40 mg per day or dexamethasone 2 to 4 mg twice daily can be used.[16] Walsh recommends dexamethasone 20 mg followed by 8 mg twice daily (0800 and 1200 to prevent steroid-induced insomnia).[17]

The following therapies have been described, but none has been studied in the palliative care setting. They are listed here as adjunctive therapy options for patients who have not responded to the above therapies.

Chlorpromazine, Promethazine

Ventafridda et al.[26] recommend the combination of chlorpromazine 25 mg (route not specified) with morphine (10 mg IM) based on experience with five patients. In addition to the morphine, chlorpromazine may control agitation and nausea and vomiting due to the morphine. Walsh[17] recommended chlorpromazine in patients whose symptoms are unrelieved by other measures. Doses recommended are 12.5 mg IV or 25 mg rectally every 4 to 12 hours. Some patients may not be able to tolerate this because of extrapyramidal effects or hypotension. Promethazine has been described as providing some relief as well.[13,16]

Inhaled Local Anesthetics

Local anesthetics (bupivicaine and lidocaine) may act to decrease J-receptor stimulation to decrease pulmonary congestion and dyspnea.

While they may cause significant bronchospasm in some people, especially those with asthma,[27] they decrease the cough reflex. Ahmedzai[2] suggests that this may be more effective for cough than for dyspnea. He also recommends that the first dose be given in a setting where bronchospasm could be quickly managed to see how the patient tolerates this therapy. This may be more effective for dyspnea caused by lymphangitis carcinomatosa.[28] Since this may decrease the gag reflex, patients should probably not eat for at least one hour[13] to several hours[28] after treatment.

Phosphodiesterase Inhibitors and Beta Sympathetic Agonists

These drugs are recommended in those patients with underlying chronic obstructive pulmonary disease. Phosphodiesterase inhibitors may increase diaphragmatic contractility and improve the efficiency of breathing.[2,13] However the clinical relevance of this has not been demonstrated. A beta-agonist agent combined with an anticholinergic agent such as ipratropium may increase bronchodilation and may be useful in older patients with chronic bronchitis.[2] These drugs may make some patients more uncomfortable by increasing heart rate, and causing tremor, agitation and anxiety.[14]

Diuretics

Diuretics are recommended in patients who may have fluid overload or congestive heart failure.[14] Furosemide 20-80 mg as needed is recommended.

Other Therapies

Other drugs may have potential in managing dyspnea based on anecdotal observations. The idea of administering respiratory "stimulants" has certain appeal, however, no pharmacologic agents are currently recommended. Agents that have been suggested include progesterone agents, nabilone (no longer available in the U.S.), doxepram, and methylphenyldate.[2,25] Progesterone agents are known to increase respiratory drive but may also cause fluid retention.[2] Nabilone (no longer available in the U.S.) may offer sedation without as much respiratory depression.[2] The side effects of these medications may increase anxiety, tremor, nervousness in patients and offset any benefits. Indomethacin may have a potential role in managing dyspnea.[13] It may be effective by preventing dyspnea caused by stimulation of the pulmonary J-receptors. Buspirone may also have a role by decreasing anxiety without the sedation caused by some of the other agents.[13]

CONCLUSION

Dyspnea is a common, distressing symptom in palliative care patients. Many factors may contribute to causing dyspnea. However, the treatment is mostly symptomatic. Opioid therapy remains the most commonly recommended. Benzodiazepines are useful for some patients, especially if anxiety is also a concomitant symptom. Other therapies that have also been used in managing dyspnea include anticholinergic agents to decrease secretions, glucocorticosteroids, chlorpromazine or promethazine, inhaled local anesthetics, asthma drugs (phosphodiasterase inhibitors and beta sympathetic agonists), and diuretics. While oxygen via a nasal cannula at about 4 liters per minute has been reported to be helpful for some patients, its use is controversial.

MEASUREMENT TOOLS

A recent report[29] summarized the tools that have been used to assess dyspnea. Most of the studies presented in Table 1 used a visual analog scale. The problem with many of these scales is they may not be sensitive enough to detect significant changes. Hay et al. compared five evaluation tools in 142 patients.[30] When an analogue and Likert type scales were used, patients reported dyspnea 32% of the time. However, when the Modified Medical Research Council Dyspnea Scale and Oxygen Cost Diagram was used, 76% and 78%, respectively, reported dyspnea with restriction of activities of living. Patient evaluations were compared to the nurse and physicians' assessments. The nurse and physician assessments were "similar"; however, the nurse agreed with the patient's assessment 47% of the time (physician 50% of the time).

Since dyspnea is multifactorial and has many components, evaluation tools that consider the patient's perception, the care giver's perception, the patient's respiratory effort and outcomes, and other factors that contribute to dyspnea, i.e., anxiety, pain, may be useful. Large variation in the classification and evaluation of dyspnea exist.

SOME OPEN RESEARCH QUESTIONS

1. Do inhaled local anesthetics have a role in managing dyspneic patients?[2]
2. When beta agonist bronchodilators are indicated, would salmeterol be a better choice because of its longer dosing interval (q12h)? MacDonald[25] posed the following questions related to managing dyspnea in the dying patient.
3. Does tolerance develop to the beneficial effects of opioids? Would rotation of the opioid drug used to treat dyspnea be beneficial?
4. Which opioid agents are the best to manage patients?
5. Do nebulized opioids offer any advantages?
6. Given that opioid-induced hypercapnia offers some symptom relief to patients, what $PaCO_2$ levels are "safe" in managing these patients?
7. Do phosphodiesterase inhibitors (theophylline, aminophylline) improve respiration?
8. Do progestational agents have any beneficial effects?
9. Does methylphenidate as a respiratory stimulant have any effect on symptom control?
10. When is oxygen indicated and beneficial for patients?

REFERENCES

1. Fishbein D. An approach to dyspnea in cancer patients. J Pain Symptom Manage 1989; 4:76-81.
2. Ahmedzai S. Palliation of respiratory symptoms. In: Doyle D, Hanks G, MacDonald N, eds. Oxford Textbook of Palliative Medicine. Oxford: Oxford University Press, 1993:349-378.
3. Reuben D. Dyspnea in terminally ill cancer patients. Chest 1986; 89:234-236.
4. Donnelly S. The symptoms of advanced cancer: Identification of clinical and research priorities by assessment of prevalence and severity. J Palliat Care 1995; 11:27-32.

5. Escalante C. Dyspnea in cancer patients. Etiology, resource utilization, and survival-implication in a managed care world. Cancer 1996; 78:1314-1319.

6. Higginson I. Measuring symptoms in terminal cancer: are pain and dyspnoea controlled? J R Soc Med 1989; 82:264-267.

7. Lynn J. Perceptions by family members of the dying experience of older and seriously ill patients. SUPPORT Investigators. Study to Understand Prognoses and Preferences for Outcomes and Risks of Treatment. Ann Intern Med 1997; 126:97-106.

8. Kemp C. Palliative care for patients with acquired immunodeficiency syndrome. Am J Hosp Palliat Care 1995; 12:14.

9. Storey P. Dyspnea. In: Storey P, ed. UNIPAC Four: Management of Selected Nonpain Symptoms in the Terminally Ill. Gainsville FL: American Academy of Hospice and Palliative Medicine, 1996:25-32.

10. Drings P. Dyspnea and cancer: Support in agonizing conditions. Support Care cancer 1997; 5:77-79.

11. Corner J. Non-pharmacological intervention for breathlessness in lung cancer. Palliat Med 1996; 10:299-305.

12. Bruera E. Effects of oxygen on dyspnoea in hypoxaemic terminal-cancer patients. Lancet 1993; 342:13-14.

13. Davis C. The therapeutics of dyspnoea. Cancer Surv 1994; 21:85-98.

14. Campbell M. Managing terminal dyspnea: caring for the patient who refuses intubation or ventilation. Dimens Crit Care Nurs 1996; 15:4-12.

15. Henteleff P. Dyspnea management: to take into the air my quiet breath. J Palliat Care 1989; 5:52-54.

16. Hsu D. Dyspnea in dying patients. Can Fam Physician 1993; 39:1635-1638.

17. Walsh D. Dyspnoea in advanced cancer. Lancet 1993; 342:450-451.

18. Cohen M. Continuous intravenous infusion of morphine for severe dyspnea. South Med J 1991; 84:229-234.

19. Dudgeon D. Dyspnea: Ethical concerns. J Palliat Care 1994; 10:48-51.

20. Bruera E. Effects of morphine on the dyspnea of terminal cancer patients. J Pain Symptom Manage 1990; 5:341-344.

21. Weatherill G. Pharmacologic symptom control during the withdrawal of life support: lessons in palliative care. AACN 1995; 6:344-351.

22. Farncombe M. Case studies outlining use of nebulized morphine for patients with end-stage chronic lung and cardiac disease. J Pain Symptom Manage 1993; 8:221-225.

23. Farncombe M. The use of nebulized opioids for breathlessness: A chart review. Palliat Med 1994; 8:306-312.

24. Farncombe M. Clinical application of nebulized opioids for treatment of dyspnoea in patients with malignant disease. Support Care Cancer 1994; 2:184-187.

25. MacDonald N. Suffering and dying in cancer patients. Research frontiers in controlling confusion, cachexia, and dyspnea. West J Med 1995; 163:278-286.

26. Ventafridda V, Spoldi E, Canno FD. Control of dyspnea in advanced cancer patients. Chest 1990; 98:1544-5.

27. McAlpine L, Thomson M. Lidocaine-induced bronchoconstriction in asthmatic patients: relation to histamine airway responsiveness and effect of preservative. Chest 1989; 96:1012-15.

28. Grey A. The nursing management of dyspnoea in palliative care. Nurs Times 1995; 91:32-35.

29. Bruera E. Subcutaneous morphine for dyspnea in cancer patients. Ann Intern Med 1993; 119:906-907.

30. van der Molen B. Dyspnoea: a study of measurement instruments for the assessment of dyspnoea and their application for patients with advanced cancer. J Adv Nurs 1995; 22:948-956.

31. Hay L, Farncombe M. McKee P. Patient, nurse and physician views of dyspnea. Canadian Nurse 1996; 93(10):26-29.

Fatigue in Palliative Care Patients

Linda S. Tyler
Arthur G. Lipman

SUMMARY. Fatigue is the most common symptom reported by patients approaching death. There is no generally accepted definition of this symptom. Some authors consider asthenia to be the same as fatigue, others do not. This monograph treats them as the same symptom. Fatigue may have multiple causes involving physical, emotional, and psychological factors. Drugs may cause or exacerbate fatigue. Identification and management of underlying causes, supportive therapy and drug therapy are described. Evaluation instruments that have been used to assess fatigue are described. Some open research questions are listed. A treatment algorithm, evidence tables and drug therapy tables are presented. *[Article copies available for a fee from The Haworth Document Delivery Service: 1-800-342-9678. E-mail address: getinfo@haworthpressinc. com <Website: http://www.haworthpressinc.com>]*

KEYWORDS. Fatigue, asthenia, weakness, palliative care, terminal care, dying, supportive care, non-pharmacological therapy, drug therapy, etiology, evidence, costs, algorithm, corticosteroids, steroids, dexamethasone, methylprednisolone, prednisone, methylphenidate, megestrol

Linda S. Tyler, PharmD, is Professor, College of Pharmacy; and Manager, Drug Information Service, Department of Pharmacy Services, University Hospitals and Clinics; University of Utah Health Sciences Center, Salt Lake City, UT.

Arthur G. Lipman, PharmD, is Professor, College of Pharmacy; Director of Clinical Pharmacology, Pain Management Center, University Hospitals and Clinics; Pain Medicine and Palliative Care Advisory Group, Huntsman Cancer Center; University of Utah Health Sciences Center, Salt Lake City, UT.

Address correspondence to: Arthur G. Lipman, PharmD, College of Pharmacy and Pain Management Center, 30 S 2000 E RM 258, University of Utah Health Sciences Center, Salt Lake City, UT 84112-5820 (E-mail: alipman@pharm.utah.edu).

[Haworth co-indexing entry note]: "Fatigue in Palliative Care Patients." Tyler, Linda S., and Arthur G. Lipman. Co-published simultaneously in *Journal of Pharmaceutical Care in Pain & Symptom Control* (Pharmaceutical Products Press, an imprint of The Haworth Press, Inc.) Vol. 8, No. 1, 2000, pp. 129-141; and: *Evidence Based Symptom Control in Palliative Care: Systematic Reviews and Validated Clinical Practice Guidelines for 15 Common Problems in Patients with Life Limiting Disease* (ed: Arthur G. Lipman, Kenneth C. Jackson II, and Linda S. Tyler) Pharmaceutical Products Press, an imprint of The Haworth Press, Inc., 2000, pp. 129-141. Single or multiple copies of this article are available for a fee from The Haworth Document Delivery Service [1-800-342-9678, 9:00 a.m. - 5:00 p.m. (EST). E-mail address: getinfo@haworthpressinc.com].

Algorithm for Managing Fatigue

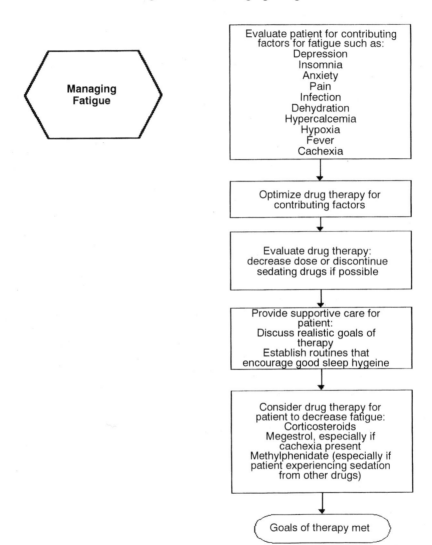

Fatigue is the most prevalent symptom in terminally ill patients. Of 100 consecutive palliative care patients, their family members, or their nurses, 83 reported weakness and 81 reported fatigue.[1] Conill et al.[2] evaluated the prevalence of symptoms in 176 terminally ill patients when the patients were first assessed by the program and compared this to the symptoms patients experienced in the last week of life. On first evaluation, weakness occurred in 77%, and in the last week of life in 82% of the patients. In another study of terminally ill cancer patients, 75% reported fatigue.[3] The report of a study of patients with advanced cancer documented 51% with weakness during a structured interview. That symptom was second only to pain which was reported by 57%.[4] Some types of cancer appear to cause a higher incidence of fatigue, i.e., lymphohematologic 75%, colorectal 68%, esophageal 64%, and lung 60%.

There is not a universal definition of fatigue.[5] Some authors distinguish between fatigue and asthenia, but for purposes of this monograph they are considered the same. Until recently, fatigue was often considered as part of the symptom complex with other diseases such as the anorexia-cachexia syndrome, depression, and anxiety. Fatigue is now recognized as a multifactorial symptom, with complex pathology, that can occur alone or in combination with other symptom complexes.

Many assessment tools have been used to identify and quantify fatigue. Some assessments of fatigue may only include a question on patient "well being" or patient activity.[6] Others ask several questions related to specific symptoms such as weakness, inability to track, difficulty starting tasks, or difficulty completing tasks.[7] Often these are part of a larger assessment tool for monitoring patient symptoms. Other tools for studying fatigue ask more extensively about the various dimensions of fatigue but are not practical to assess patients on a routine basis.[8-10] Some authors have tried to adapt these tools to clinical practice, but found in simplifying the tools, they were unable to assess some of the complexities of fatigue.[11] Richardson,[12] Stone et al.[13] and Varricchio[14] reviewed several of the instruments used to assess fatigue.

Fatigue encompasses physical, emotional, and psychological components. Yet little is known about the mechanisms of fatigue and even less about the management. Several authors have reviewed fatigue in general,[15] fatigue in cancer patients,[9,13,16-18] and fatigue in palliative care patients.[19-21] The diagnosis of fatigue is based on the patient's report of the symptom. Some patients may voluntarily report fatigue. But often it goes unrecognized unless the practitioner specifically asks. Coyle et al.[22] evaluated the spontaneous report of symptoms in 90 patients who were followed by a supportive care program. Fifty-eight percent reported fatigue and 43% weakness 4 weeks prior to death. Within the week prior to death, 52% reported fatigue and 49% reported weakness. Fatigue was the most prevalent symptom in these patients. No attempt was made to elicit additional information from patients after asking in general how they felt.

Patients may be reluctant to mention fatigue. They may feel that their care givers may not give their complaint the importance they would like. From the care giver's perspective, fatigue is not easily addressed and often there is little to offer the patient. This may give the patient the impression that fatigue is not worth addressing. Yet fatigue may interfere with patients' ability to make end of life plans and decisions.

Several strategies may be considered to manage fatigue. The first step is to assess the patient and identify any other symptoms or diseases that may contribute to fatigue. Some of these conditions might be addressed to decrease the fatigue. Depression and anxiety can cause fatigue. If therapy for those symptoms has been instituted, it should be optimized. Cachexia and lack of sleep also contribute to fatigue. Patients with pain often also have fatigue. Opioids used to treat pain can also contribute to fatigue, especially in the first week after initiation of pharmacotherapy, dose escalation, and when the patient is experiencing significant sedation. Patients often develop tolerance to the opioid-induced sedation effects after about a week on stable doses. Other drugs that cause sedation may worsen patients' fatigue. When possible these drugs should be decreased in dose or discontinued. Dehydration also causes fatigue. This can often be managed with oral hydration.

Other causes of fatigue may not be appropriate or practical to address in palliative care. For example, anemia is a common cause of fatigue. However, the treatment for anemia (blood transfusions or epoetin) is very expensive and loses effect with repeated use. Thus it has little usefulness in palliative care. However, a transfusion may be indicated in palliative care when it provides the needed strength for the patient to attend an important event such as a family wedding or grandchild's graduation. Infections also cause fatigue. Controversy exists about the role of exercise. For many patients, some activity helps decrease fatigue; for others, it may exacerbate the complaint. Metabolic diseases that have been associated with fatigue include malnutrition, hypercalcemia, adrenal insufficiency, hypoxia and hypothyroidism.

EVALUATE THE CAUSES OF FATIGUE

Fatigue is associated with many other disease states and symptoms. The patient should be thoroughly evaluated for any of the following:

- Depression
- Insomnia
- Anxiety
- Pain
- Infection
- Fever
- Dehydration
- Anorexia or cachexia
- Hypercalcemia
- Hypoxia
- Drugs, especially those that may cause CNS depression

TREAT THE UNDERLYING CAUSE OR CONTRIBUTOR TO FATIGUE WHEN POSSIBLE

When a potential cause of fatigue is identified, the clinician must decide whether to treat the underlying disease or address contributing cause. Patients' fatigue often lessens after their therapy for pain, fever, depression, insomnia, and anxiety are optimized. Many patients experience increased energy and sense of well being when their cachexia is treated. If the patient is taking any drugs that may contribute to fatigue, dose decreases or discontinuation should be considered. Dehydration should be treated.

IMPLEMENT SUPPORTIVE THERAPY

Caregivers should discuss fatigue with patients and set realistic goals. For the patient, knowing what to expect will make it easier to manage. It is important for the patient to know that you understand how fatigue is affecting them. Several non-pharmacologic strategies may be helpful.[16,19] One is to establish routines that reinforce good sleep hygiene principles. These includes using a set bedtime and wake-up time, and incorporating rest periods during the day. Frequent napping may contribute to insomnia and fatigue in some patients. Scheduled rest periods can be used. Some patients, however, may need additional sleep time. Eliminate or decrease unnecessary activities (such as housework) or activities that drain the patient's energy. No data are available that assess non-pharmacologic interventions in the palliative care patient.

TREAT FATIGUE PHARMACOLOGICALLY

Pharmacologic interventions may benefit some patients. Table 1 summarizes the evidence on drug therapy for managing fatigue. A universal limitation of all these studies was that they were not designed to assess fatigue specifically, i.e., fatigue was not the primary endpoint. These studies involved relatively small numbers of patients.

Corticosteroids have been beneficial and should be considered for many patients. No randomized, double-blind studies were designed with fatigue as the primary endpoint.[23-27] Corticosteroids demonstrated improvements in patients' overall sense of well-being and appetite.

Megestrol acetate has demonstrated some benefit in cancer patients with demonstrated weight loss.[28-30] While definitions vary between the studies, each study selected patients with demonstrated weight loss in the previous month. Megestrol acetate resulted in weight gain, increased appetite, and increased sense of well-being while patients were taking the drug and the effect was sustained in patients who took the drug for a longer time. In managing fatigue, megestrol has only been studied in those patients who also have cachexia.

The optimal initial dose is not known. Loprinzi[31] evaluated four doses of megestrol–60, 480, 800, and 1,280 mg–and found the greatest effect on weight gain with the 800 mg dose. No increased efficacy was noted at the higher dose. At the lower doses, a clear dose response relationship exists, the higher the dose, the greater the weight gain. However, this study did not assess fatigue. Other authors have demonstrated weight gain at doses of 160 to 320 mg.[29] If patients are going

TABLE 1. Drug Therapy for Managing Fatigue in Palliative Care–Evidence Tables

Reference	Study Design	n	Intervention	Results	Level of Evidence	Comments
Corticosteroids						
Moertel (1974)[23]	Randomized double-blind	116	Patients with unresectable gastrointestinal adenocarcinoma received placebo, dexamethasone 0.75 mg po qid, or dexamethasone 1.5 mg po qid. Therapy continued until patients died or could not take oral drugs.	Patients on dexamethasone compared to placebo reported improved strength at 2 weeks (26% vs. 15%) and 4 weeks (34% vs. 13%). Results were not statistically significant. Survival was similar to placebo.	II	Did not specifically address fatigue.
Bruera (1985)[27]	Randomized double-blind	40	Patients who were terminally ill were randomized to receive methylprednisolone 16 mg po bid or placebo for 5 days, then crossed over to 5 days of the alternate therapy after a 3 day washout interval. After the crossover, all patients received 16 mg bid me hylprednisolone.	31 patients completed the trial. Patients who received methylprednisolone demonstrated significant improvement in pain, depression, appetite, activity and food consumption. No change was noted on anxiety and performance status. 61% of patients reported better activity level on methylprednisolone compared to 16% who were better on placebo and 23% who reported no difference.	II	Did not specifically address fatigue, but did access activity and performance status. Small numbers of patients studied. Treatment with the drug was of short duration.
Robustelli Della Cuna (1989)[25]	Placebo controlled multicenter study	403	Patients with preterminal cancer were randomized to receive 125 mg per day of methylprednisolone sodium succinate iv (n = 207) or placebo (n = 196) for 8 weeks.	Quality of life was assessed using the Nurses Observational Scale for Inpatient Evaluation (NOSIE), Linear Analogue Self Assessment (LASA) scale, and Physician's Global Evaluation Scale. Patients receiving methylprednisolone demonstrated significantly improved scores on NOSIE. On the LASA, significant improvement was noted in pain, appetite, vomiting and well-being scores. Using the physician's evaluation, the therapeutic effect of methylprednisolone was evaluated as good to excellent in 42% of patients compared to 21% on placebo. The survival rate was similar in male patients, but female patients on methylprednisolone showed a statistically significant better survival rate.	II	Symptoms related to fatigue was assessed as part of larger tool.

TABLE 1 (continued)

Reference	Study Design	n	Intervention	Results	Level of Evidence	Comments
Popicia (1989)[24]	Randomized double-blind	173	Female cancer patients who were terminally ill received methylprednisolone 125 mg IV qd or placebo for 56 days.	Used LASA assessment. Patients on methylprednisolone demonstrated significantly improved quality of life, including increased appetite, sense of well-being.	II	Did not specifically address fatigue. Groups demonstrated equal mortality and adverse effects.
Twycross (1985)[26]	Randomized double-blind	27	Patients with terminal cancer received prednisolone 10 mg once then 5 mg po tid (n = 16) versus placebo (n = 11) for 7 days	prednisolone improved mood, sleep, and appetite; the difference was not significant.	II	Did not specifically address fatigue. Small number of patients.
Megestrol Acetate (Megace)						
Oster (1994)[28]	Randomized double-blind	100	Patients with AIDS and cachexia were randomized to receive megestrol acetate 800 mg per day or placebo PO for 12 weeks.	Patients receiving megestrol acetate demonstrated significant weight gain (mean = 4.77 kg, CI95 = 2.06-7.48kg) and increased sense of well-being.	II	Did not specifically address fatigue.
Gebbia (1996)[29]	Randomized double-blind	122	Cancer patients with cachexia or anorexia were randomized to receive megestrol acetate 160 mg po qd or 160 mg po q12h. Patients were evaluated every 2 weeks. If after one month of therapy weight and appetite did not increase, the dose was increased to 320 or 480 mg per day, respectively.	Increased weight was noted in 27% vs. 40% of patients at the lower vs. higher doses respectively after 15 days of therapy. After dosage increases, 18% of 320 mg group and 10% of the 480 mg group gained weight. Increased appetite was reported in 36% and 20% of patients respectively. Energy improved in 16(39%) of the 41 with low energy at the start of the study in the lower dose group and 16 (46%) of 35 in the higher dose. Differences were not statistically significant.	I	Did not specifically address fatigue. Authors recommend starting dose of 160 mg per day with increases if no response. Patient response was noted at 2 weeks. This was not a placebo controlled trial.

Bruera (1990)[30]	Randomized double-blind, cross-over	40	Malnourished patients with advanced tumors, non hormone response, receiving no antineoplastic therapy, were randomized to receive megestrol acetate 480 mg per day or placebo for 7 days then crossed-over to the alternative therapy.	Patients demonstrated statistically significant improvement in subjective energy level while on megestrol acetate compared to placebo. No significant difference in well-being noted.	II	Did not specifically address fatigue.

Methylphenidate (Ritalin)

Bruera (1987)[32]	Randomized, double-blind, cross-over	32	Patients with chronic pain due to advanced cancer received either methylphenidate 10 mg with breakfast and 5 mg with lunch for 3 days or placebo. They were then crossed over to the alternative therapy.	28 patients completed trial. Found no significant difference in sensation of well being. A statistically significant difference was noted in improvement of activity between methylphenidate and placebo.	II	This trial was designed to assess impact of therapy on patients' pain. It did not assess fatigue directly.

Key to Level of Evidence classification:

Level I   Randomized trials with low false-positive (alpha) and low false-negative (beta errors); high power
Level II   Randomized trials with high false-positive (alpha) and/or high false-negative (beta errors); low power
Level III   Nonrandomized concurrent cohort comparisons between contemporaneous patients who did and did not receive a given intervention
Level IV   Nonrandomized historical cohort comparisons between current patients who did receive the intervention and patients (from the same institution or from the literature) who did not
Level V   Case series without control subjects

TABLE 2. Drug Therapy for Managing Fatigue in Palliative Care

Drug Therapy	Indications for Use	Dosing Regimen	AWP per Day of Therapy
Corticosteroids	Clinical trials report that patients demonstrate increased appetite and sense of well-being. May be especially useful in patients who have other reasons to take corticosteroids, such as bone pain or bronchospasm.	Dexamethasone 4 mg po bid or tid (available as 0.5 mg/5mL solution) 2-4 mg po bid or tid (tablets) 2-4 mg po bid or tid (Available as 0.5 m/5 mL elixir) Prednisone 10-20 mg po qd or bid Methylprednisolone 16 mg po bid Methylprednisolone sodium succinate 125mg IV qd	$1.16-1.75 $1.90-5.70 $0.03-0.13 $1.83
Megestrol acetate (Megace)	Clinical trials demonstrate that patients have increased weight gain, appetite, and sense of well-being. Data on its use is in patients who have cachexia.	160-800 mg po daily	$3.42-17.00 $1.76-8.80
Methylphenidate (Ritalin)	Probably most useful in patients experiencing sedation secondary to pain medications.	10 mg at breakfast, 5 mg at lunch	

to respond to therapy, a response is observed within 2 weeks. If patients do not respond to a given dose, the dose may be increased with many patients responding to the increased dose.

Some authors recommend methylphenidate or dextroamphetamine,[19] especially for patients who may have increased fatigue because of CNS active drugs. However, little evidence supports this use. Bruera et al.[32] compared the effect of methylphenidate 10 mg at breakfast, 5 mg at lunch, to placebo in a randomized, double-blind cross-over trial in 32 patients with pain related to the presence of a tumor. Patients receiving methylphenidate demonstrated a statistically significant increase in activity, However the purpose of the study was to assess pain intensity, which also decreased with methylphendiate.

SOME OPEN RESEARCH QUESTIONS

1. What would be the best way to assess fatigue in a clinical setting?
2. What patients would benefit best from corticosteroids or megestrol therapy?
3. What is the role of CNS stimulant drugs in managing fatigue?

REFERENCES

1. Ng K, von Gunten CF. Symptoms and attitudes of 100 consecutive patients admitted to an acute hospice/palliative care unit. J Pain Symptom Manage. 1998; 16:307 315.

2. Conill C, Veiger E, Henriquez I, et al. Symptom prevalence in the last week of life. J Pain Symptom Manage. 1997;14:328-331.

3. Bruera E, MacDonald RN. Overwhelming fatigue in advanced cancer. Amer J Nursing. 1988:99-100.

4. Vainio A, Auvinen A. Prevalence of symptoms among patients with advanced cancer: An International collaborative study. J Pain Symptom Manage. 1996;12:3-10.

5. Portenoy RK. Introduction: Asthenia: definitions and dimensions. In: Bruera E, Portenoy RK, eds. Topics in Palliative Care. New York Oxford: Oxford University Press; 1998:167-169.

6. Bruera E, Kuehn N, Miller M, et al. The Edmonton symptom assessment system (ESAS): A simple method for the assessment of palliative care patients. J Palliative Care. 1991;7:6-9.

7. Bliss JM, Robertson B, Selby PJ. The impact of nausea and vomiting upon quality of life measures. Br J Cancer Suppl. 1992;66:314-323.

8. Smets E, Garssen B, Bonke B, de Haes J. The multidimensional fatigue inventory: Psychometric qualities of an instrument to assess fatigue. J Psychomsom Res. 1995;39:315-329.

9. Smets E, Garssen B, de Haes J. Application of the multidimensional fatigue inventory in cancer patients receiving radiotherapy. Br J Cancer. 1996;73:241-245.

10. Yellen SB, Cella DF, Webster K, Blendowski C, Kaplan E. Measuring fatigue and other anemia-related symptoms with the functional assessment of cancer therapy (FACT) measurement system. J Pain Symptom Manage. 1997;13:63-74.

11. Schneider RA. Reliability and validity of the multidimensional fatigue inventory (MFI-20) and the rhoten fatigue scale among rural cancer outpatients. Cancer Nursing. 1998;21:370-373.

12. Richardson A. Measuring fatigue in patients with cancer. Support Care Cancer. 1998;6:94-100.

13. Stone P, Richards M, Hardy J. Fatigue in patients with cancer. Europ Jf Cancer. 1998;34:1670-1676.

14. Varricchio CG. Selecting a tool for measuring fatigue. Oncology Nursing Forum. 1985;12:122-127.

15. von Hoff DP. Asthenia: Incidence, etiology, pathophysiology, and treatment. Cancer Therapeutics. 1998;1:184-197.

16. Miaskowski C, Portenoy RK. Update on the assessment and management of cancer-related fatigue. Principles and Practice of Supportive Oncology Updates. 1998;1:1-10.

17. Irvine DM, Vincent L, Bubela N, Thompson L, Graydon J. A critical appraisal of the research literature investigating fatigue in the individual with cancer. Cancer Nursing. 1991;14:188-199.

18. Winningham ML, Nail LM, Burke MB, et al. Fatigue and the cancer experience: The state of the knowledge. Oncology Nursing Forum. 1994;21:23-36.

19. Neuenschwander H, Bruera E. Asthenia. In: Doyle D, Hanks GWC, MacDonald N, eds. Oxford Textbook of Palliative Medicine. Oxford New York Tokyo: Oxford University Press; 1998:573-581.

20. Neuenschwander H, Bruera E. Pathophysiology of cancer asthenia. In: Bruera E, Portenoy RK, eds. Topics in Palliative Care. Volume 1, New York Oxford: Oxford University Press; 1998:171-181.

21. Cleary JF. The reversible causes of asthenia in cancer patients. In: Bruera E, Portenoy RK, eds. Topics in Palliative Care, Volume 1, New York Oxford: Oxford University Press; 1998:183-202.

22. Coyle N, Adelhardt J, Foley KM, Portenoy RK. Character of terminal illness in the advanced cancer patient: pain and other symptoms during the last four weeks of life. J Pain Symptom Manage. 1990;5:83-93.

23. Moertel CG, Schutt AJ, Reitemeier RJ, Hahn RG. Corticosteroid therapy of preterminal gastrointestinal cancer. Cancer. 1974;33:1607-1609.

24. Popiela T, Lucchi R, Giongo F. Methylprednisolone as palliative therapy for female terminal cancer patients. Eur J Cancer Clin Oncol. 1989;25:1823-1829.

25. Robustelli Della Cuna G, Pellegrini A, Piazzi M. Effect of methylprednisolone sodium succinate on quality of life in preterminal cancer patients: a placebo-controlled, multicenter study. Eur J Cancer Clin Oncol. 1989;25:1817-1821.

26. Twycross RG, Guppy D. Prednisolone in terminal breast and bronchogenic cancer. Practitioner. 1985;229:57-59.

27. Bruera E, Roca E, Cedaro L, Carraro S, Chacon R. Action of oral methylprednisolone in terminal cancer patients: a prospective randomized double-blind study. Cancer Treat Rep. 1985;69:751-754.

28. Oster MH, Enders SR, Samuels SJ, et al. Megestrol acetate in patients with AIDS and cachexia. Ann Int Med. 1994;121:400-408.

29. Gebbia V, Testa A, Gebbia N. Prospective randomised trial of two dose levels of megestrol acetate in the management of anorexia-cachexia syndrome in patients with metastatic cancer. Br J Cancer. 1996;73:1576-1580.

30. Bruera E, Macmillan K, Kuehn N, Hanson J, MacDonald RN. A controlled trial of megestrol acetate on appetite, caloric intake, nutritional status, and other symptoms in patients with advanced cancer. Cancer. 1990;66:1279-1282.

31. Loprinzi CL, Schaid DJ, Dose AM, Burnham NL, Jens. Body-composition changes in patients who gain weight while receiving megestrol acetate. J Clin Oncol. 1993;11:152-154.

32. Bruera E, Chadwick S, Brennels C, Hanson J, MacDonald RN. Methylphenidate associated with narcotics for the treatment of cancer pain. Cancer Treat Rep. 1987;71:67-70.

Oral Mucosal Problems
in Palliative Care Patients

Kenneth C. Jackson II
Mark S. Chambers

SUMMARY. Oral mucosal damage due to stomatitis and mucositis in palliative care patients is described. Causes and general supportive measures are discussed. Drugs associated with xerostomia are listed. Disease and drug induced changes in taste are addressed. Treatments used for oral mucosal damage are described. Evaluation instruments that have been used to assess oral mucosal damage are described. Some open research questions are listed. A prevention algorithm, a treatment algorithm and therapy tables are presented. *[Article copies available for a fee from The Haworth Document Delivery Service: 1-800-342-9678. E-mail address: getinfo@haworthpressinc.com <Website: http://www.haworthpressinc.com>]*

KEYWORDS. Mucosa, oral, mucositis, stomatitis, damage, dysgeusia, xerostomia, dry mouth, prevention, palliative care, terminal care, dying, supportive care, drug therapy, non-pharmacological therapy, etiology, evidence, costs, algorithm, radiotherapy, chemotherapy, hygiene, allopurinol, antibiotics, azelastine, chamomile, chlorhexidine, colony-stimulating factors, cryotherapy, glutamine, helium-neon laser treatment, immune globulin, non-steroidal anti-inflammatory drugs, pentoxyphylline, povidone-iodine, propantheline, prostaglandins, sucralfate, cryotherapy

Kenneth C. Jackson II, PharmD, is Manager of Clinical Pharmacy Services, St. Dominic-Jackson Memorial Hospital; and Clinical Assistant Professor, University of Mississippi School of Pharmacy, Jackson, MS.

Mark S. Chambers, DMD, MS, is Associate Professor, Department of Dental Oncology, University of Texas M.D. Anderson Cancer Center, Houston, TX.

Address correspondence to: Arthur G. Lipman, PharmD, College of Pharmacy and Pain Management Center, 30 S 2000 E RM 258, University of Utah Health Sciences Center, Salt Lake City, UT 84112-5820 (E-mail: alipman@pharm.utah.edu).

[Haworth co-indexing entry note]: "Oral Mucosal Problems in Palliative Care Patients." Jackson, Kenneth C. II, and Mark S. Chambers. Co-published simultaneously in *Journal of Pharmaceutical Care in Pain & Symptom Control* (Pharmaceutical Products Press, an imprint of The Haworth Press, Inc.) Vol. 8, No. 1, 2000, pp. 143-161; and: *Evidence Based Symptom Control in Palliative Care: Systematic Reviews and Validated Clinical Practice Guidelines for 15 Common Problems in Patients with Life Limiting Disease* (ed: Arthur G. Lipman, Kenneth C. Jackson II, and Linda S. Tyler) Pharmaceutical Products Press, an imprint of The Haworth Press, Inc., 2000, pp. 143-161. Single or multiple copies of this article are available for a fee from The Haworth Document Delivery Service [1-800-342-9678, 9:00 a.m. - 5:00 p.m. (EST). E mail address: getinfo@haworthpressinc.com].

143

Algorithm for Mucositis Prevention

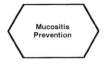

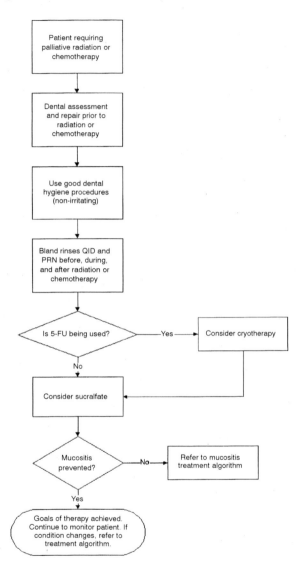

Algorithm for Mucositis Treatment

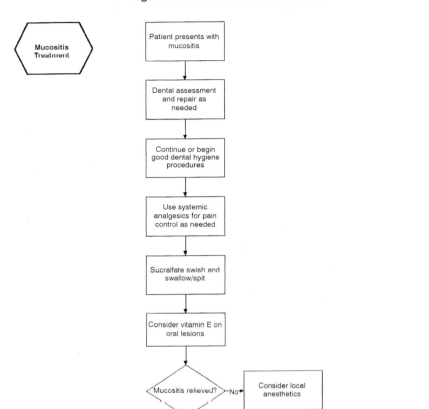

Oral mucositis is a pathological condition of the mucous membrane of the oral cavity. The mouth is the portal of entry and place of mastication for food and it contains taste organs. Saliva produced in the oral cavity not only lubricates food to facilitate swallowing, but also contains buffers, enzymes, and antimicrobial components. It is lined throughout by the mucous membrane, a term that denotes the lining of any body cavity that communicates with the outside.

Dry mouth, mucositis, and subsequent damage in the oral mucosa have profound implications in terminally ill patients. As many as 70% of hospice patients suffer from xerostomia.[1] A recent analysis revealed that oral side effects occurred with 79% of commonly prescribed medications.[2] Xerostomia was the most problematic of the oral side effects, occurring in 80.5% of these cases. Stomatitis, although not as frequent (33.9%), occurred at a rate that should concern. Mucositis occurs in 40% to 70% of patients undergoing chemotherapy or radiotherapy.[3]

EVIDENCE

There is no standard effective therapy for the treatment or prevention of oral mucositis. Many investigators have attempted to define effective treatment for mucositis. A review of mucositis trials in the treatment for cure cancer population has been published elsewhere.[4] To date no trials have been conducted in terminally ill patients. Due to the differences in these populations, extrapolation of these data to the terminally ill population presents many difficulties.

Mucositis management research can be divided into two categories: prevention and treatment. Modalities studied for mucositis prevention include aggressive oral hygiene, allopurinol, antibiotics, azelastine, chamomile, chlorhexidine, colony-stimulating factors, cryotherapy, glutamine, helium-neon laser treatment, immune globulin, non-steroidal anti-inflammatory drugs, pentoxyphylline, povidone iodine, propantheline, prostaglandins, and sucralfate. Cryotherapy and aggressive oral hygiene therapy are the preventative measures that present the least discomfort to patients while providing some efficacy in preventing mucositis.[4]

Many therapies have been studied for the treatment of mucositis including anesthetics, capsaicin, chamomile, chlorhexidine, cryotherapy, mesalamine, non-steroidal medications, opioids, sucralfate, tetrachlorodecaoxide, and vitamin E. Most anti-inflammatory, anesthetic, and topical coating agents known have also been studied. Topical agents such as sucralfate and vitamin E may offer some relief to areas with structural compromise. Pain relief provided by capsaicin or local anesthetics, especially in novel delivery systems, may provide limited pain relief to patients with mucositis. Opioids remain the gold standard for alleviation of pain, yet they offer little in the way of disease modification. The role of aggressive therapies such as immune globulin, colony stimulating factors, and neon-helium laser treatment remain unclear in all populations, especially the terminally ill patient subset.

The presence of a healthy mouth prior to radiotherapy or chemotherapy reduces a patient's risk of post-treatment complications. Oral complications in cancer patients receiving cytotoxic therapy can lead to systemic involvement.[5,6] The oral cavity should be evaluated in all advanced disease patients, regardless of their primary diagnosis. Preventing and treating oral complications seen in this population is important. Anticipating primary and secondary mucosal insults and recognizing oral complications promptly can decrease the incidence of complications or ameliorate their morbid effects. A thorough oral examination and treatment following established guidelines can correct potential clinical and radiographic pathology before this occurs.[7-9]

The general term stomatitis can be applied when mucosal integrity has been lost due to local trauma, i.e., biting, denture irritation, or infection.[10] Treatment usually consists of smoothing rough teeth, prescribing mucosal toothguards, and stressing to the patient the importance of a soft diet in order to decrease functional irritation and trauma.[8-10] Prostheses can cause or exacerbate stomatitis by producing traumatic wounds as well as providing a sanctuary for microorganisms by shielding the mucosa from oral hygiene or appropriate topical medication rinses.[11] In addition, dentures can hold the microbes in close proximity to any lesion that may develop under the dentures. Stomatitis often is preventable or can be corrected with dental or antimicrobial treatment.

Mucositis is the cytotoxic reaction of the oral mucosal tissues to chemotherapy or radiotherapy. The differential diagnosis should first rule out other factors, e.g., infection, trauma, factitious injury. Mucosal reactions identified incorrectly can cause effective therapy to be delayed, chemotherapy dosage to be reduced, or chemotherapy or radiotherapy to be completely discontinued. Thus, oral care should include microorganism assays by culture to evaluate the incidence of mucositis versus infection.[8,9] The patient should be urged to report any mucosal changes or increased sensitivity.

Considerable interpatient variability exists in the tolerance to chemotherapy regimens and the development of mucositis. There are the chemotherapy agents that, depending on the dosage and duration, will produce mucositis, i.e., antimetabolites, antibiotics, and to a lesser degree, alkylating agents and vinca alkaloids. However, from what has been observed, any agent given at an intensified dose or for sufficient duration will produce direct or secondary mucosal toxicities that will be dose-limiting for therapy.[7,12] Treatment factors that influence the frequency and severity of oral mucositis induced by chemotherapy include the drug used, dose, administration schedule, and concurrent radiotherapy.[13] It is important to recognize the temporal the relationship between the administration of chemotherapy and any mucosal reactions.

Therapeutic administration of ionizing radiation to the head and neck produces a number of oral changes, including mucosal thinning, salivary gland atrophy, vascular fibrosis, and damage to the taste buds. These complications are generally of two types: acute, e.g., treatment-related mucositis, infectious stomatitis, and long-term, e.g., xerostomia, dental decay, trismus, hypovascularity, osteoradionecrosis. The severity of mucositis induced by radiation therapy depends on a number of factors including the administered dose, the dose fraction, the volume of tissue radiated, type of radiation given, and administration of a concomitant boost.[13,14] Other factors that may contribute to the severity of mucositis include smoking, over-the-counter mouthwashes, collagen vascular disease, and HIV infection.[13]

Mucositis can be an acute clinical manifestation of radiation toxicity to the rapidly proliferating cells in the basal regions of the epithelium.[13] Decreased cell regeneration leads to epithelial atrophy and mucosal thinning. All intraoral sites may be affected, although nonkeratinized surfaces are most severely affected. Erythema is the initial manifestation, followed by the development of white desquamative patches that are painful on contact. Epithelial sloughing and fibrinous exudate lead to the formation of a pseudomembrane and ulceration and represent a more marked form of mucositis.[13] Epithelial cell loss also results in the exposure of the richly innervated underlying connective tissue stroma, which contributes to the pain associated with the more severe forms of mucositis. Healing occurs, on average, 3-4 weeks after completion of conventionally fractionated radiotherapy.

Irradiation can permanently destroy cellular elements of bone, which can limit the potential for wound maintenance and the ability to heal after a traumatic event.[9,15] Furthermore, the risk of complications following trauma or oral surgical procedures in an irradiated field can be highly significant, although some authors claim this risk is low up to a predetermined threshold of irradiation.[16-18] For these reasons, elective oral surgical procedures such as extractions and soft tissue surgery are contraindicated within an irradiated field.[9,19] However, nonsurgical dental work that can be safely done include routine restorative procedures, oral prophylaxis, radiography, and endodontic and prosthodontic procedures.

Xerostomia, or dry mouth, is oral dryness caused by a lack of normal salivary secretion due either to reduction in salivary flow or alteration of salivary composition. Xerostomia can result from medications or may be a sign of poor nutritional status. Untreated, xerostomia can compromise the integrity of the oral mucosa and place patients at risk for further complications. Such a condition can prolong or intensify the process of mucosal erosion and ulceration. Saliva is a complex fluid consisting of electrolytes, proteins, glycoproteins, and lipids. Many studies have shown that saliva plays a significant role in maintaining the integrity of the teeth and oral mucosa.[20] Individuals who have lost the protective qualities of saliva can exhibit innumerable problems with their teeth and oral mucosa.[21] These can include increased dental caries, dehydration of the mucosa, and oral infections that will lead to great discomfort and difficulty in chewing, swallowing, and speaking.

Pharmacologic agents, radiotherapy to the head and neck, and surgery that involves a major salivary gland are the medical therapies that most commonly interfere with salivary function. Radiation therapy for head and neck cancer causes salivary gland damage and oral mucosal insult in most patients and is an important cause of xerostomia and mucositis. Chemotherapeutic agents are cytotoxic, and their use often directly and adversely affects the rapidly replicating oral mucosa. Cytotoxicity produces thinning, denudation, and ulceration of the buccal mucosa, tongue, gingivae, and pharynx. Many drugs can cause or exacerbate xerostomia and as a result intensify the degree of mucositis through their actions.

NON-CANCER PATIENTS

The majority of terminally ill patients in hospice care have a cancer diagnoses. However many patients have diagnoses that are unrelated to cancer. While these patients usually do not receive chemotherapy or radiotherapy, they are still at risk for developing complications in their oral cavity. It is important to closely monitor these patients' oral health and refer them for dental consultation when indicated. Additionally, this patient population is still at risk for the oral adverse effects of many medications.

Many hospice patients may present with preexisting oral pathology that can adversely impact dental health including broken or rough teeth, gingivitis, ill fitting appliances or prostheses, and periodontal disease. These conditions can inflict local trauma and serve as a nidus for infection. Appropriate dental evaluation and treatment is necessary to avoid these complications, as well as the associated pain and discomfort.

For oral complication pain, analgesics, especially opioids, should be instituted if they are not already part of the patient's therapeutic regimen. When analgesic therapy is already in place, dose escalation may be warranted. Unfortunately, a number of medications, including opioids, used in palliative care may cause or exacerbate xerostomia. This should not deter clinicians from using these medications, especially for control of pain and resulting anxiety.

Prevention of mucositis and other forms of oral pathology should be a primary concern to those caring for terminally ill patients. Prophylaxis is especially important for patients undergoing radiotherapy of the head and neck region and patients receiving certain chemotherapeutic regimens. Many patients develop oral disease despite prophylaxis and require active treatment of their oral pathology. Patients who are non-compliant with preventative measures will become candidates for active treatment.

OTHER ORAL COMPLICATIONS

A number of complications can be seen in the oral cavity of terminally ill patients. Many patients may have disease or damage to the periodontal region that predates their terminal illness. Additionally, patients may present with ongoing disease that was neglected during prior treatment phases of their illness. Problems in the oral cavity can place patients at risk for systemic complications. Examples of problems with the oral cavity, and systemic complications include:[1,3,22-25]

Local and Systemic Complications of Oral Pathology

- Caries
- Dysgeusia and halitosis
- Dysphagia
- Infection (local or systemic; bacterial or fungal)
- Impaired hydration or nutritional status
- Mucositis
- Muscle trismus (radiation induced)
- Oral hemorrhage
- Osteoradionecrosis
- Pain
- Sialorrhea (excessive salivation)
- Structural damage to oral mucosa
- Xerostomia (dry mouth)
- Ulcers (drug-induced, neutropenic, traumatic, viral)

MEDICATIONS AND ORAL COMPLICATIONS

Medication administration always carries the risk of producing untoward effects in patients. Complications from medications in the oral cavity include dysgeusia, mucositis, and xerostomia.[1,3,15,22,24,26] Clinicians should consider the patient's entire medication regimen for possible offending agents.

XEROSTOMIA

More than 250 drugs may cause xerostomia.[27,28] As drug regimens increase in number, so do the complaints of dry mouth.[2,27] Several drug classes are problematic in palliative care, most commonly the opioids. Additionally, certain anticonvulsants, antidepressants, antiemetics, benzodiazepines, diuretics, and neuroleptics may cause xerostomia.

Medications Known to Cause Xerostomia[1,3,22,24,25,27-31]	
Class	*Selected Examples*
Opioids	morphine, methadone, oxycodone, fentanyl
Ace inhibitors	enalapril, lisinopril
Anticonvulsants	carbamazepine
Antidepressants	amitriptyline, desipramine, doxepin, fluoxetine, sertraline
Anti-emetics	metoclopramide
Anti-histamines	diphenhydramine, chlorpheniramine
Benzodiazepines	alprazolam, diazepam, triazolam
Beta blockers	propranolol, metoprolol
Calcium channel blockers	nifedipine
Cardiac glycosides	digoxin
Diuretics	furosemide, hydrochlorothiazide, sprironolactone
Neuroleptics	chlorpromazine, thioridazine
NSAIDs	ibuprofen

A variety of therapeutic and palliative agents have been used to manage the sequelae associated with salivary gland dysfunction. Selection of an adequate management regimen for a particular patient with xerostomia should be based on reports of discomfort or dysfunction, presence of oral changes, and presence of any additional factors that compromise oral health.[15] There can be a poor correlation between subjective reports and actual gland function as well as a large variation in degrees of salivary function found with xerostomia.

Treatment is aimed initially at restoring the flow of saliva using mechanical means and taste stimulants or systemic salivary gland stimulants (sialogogues). Artificial saliva substitutes and mouth wetting agents may be used, although most provide only short-term relief of symptoms and can irritate already sensitive oral tissues in the long term. Currently, extrinsic saliva substitutes are divided into two groups based upon the presence or absence of natural mucins. Sialogogues include the widely used stimulant pilocarpine. Individuals who suffer from the oral sequelae associated with salivary gland dysfunction and mucositis present a special challenge to clinicians in terms of early diagnosis, prevention, and initiation of competent treatment.[15,21]

Changes in salivary flow induced by radiation are worrisome because saliva protects the oral mucosa from dehydration and assists in the mechanical lavage of food and microbial debris from the oral cavity.[32] To avoid oral infections that may arise from radiation therapy, the patient must frequently rinse the oral cavity to reduce the number of oral microorganisms and to maintain mucosal hydration.[33] When the salivary glands are involved in a radiation field, the daily use of a fluoride gel is necessary to prevent caries due to the decrease in saliva.

DYSGEUSIA

Dysgeusia due to medications is under appreciated. Dysgeusia has been reported to occur as a side effect in as many as 24.5% of the top 200 prescribed medications.[2] While dysgeusia may not directly harm patients, the impact of this disorder should not be minimized. In addition to the obvious discomfort associated with poor taste, dysgeusia can impact patient compliance and nutritional status. Medications that cause adverse taste alterations should be eliminated when possible. When this is not possible, attempts at masking the taste or providing other means of alleviating the taste should be pursued. The following is a selected list of agents that may be implicated in dysgeusia.

Medications Implicated in Dysgeusia[2,3]	
Class	*Selected Examples*
ACE inhibitors	captopril, enalapril
Antibiotics	cephlasporins, ciprofloxacin, clarithromycin, norfloxacin, ofloxacin, penicillin
Antidepressants	amitriptyline, nortriptyline, sertraline
Antihyperlipidemics	gemfibrozil, lovastatin
Antiparkinsonian	carbidopa/levodopa
Antiviral	acyclovir
Benzodiazepines	alprazolam, diazepam, flurazepam, lorazepam, triazolam
Bronchodialators	albuterol
Calcium channel blockers	diltiazem, nifedipine
Antihypertensives	propranolol, guanfacine
H$_2$ blockers	famotidine
Diuretics	triamterene/hydrochlorothiazide
Hormonal agent	tamoxifen
Mast cell stabilizers	cromolyn
Muscle relaxants	cyclobenzaprine
Nicotine replacement	nicotine polacrilex (Nicorette), topical nicotine
Opioids	codeine, oxycodone, propoxyphene
Proton pump inhibitors	omeprazole
NSAIDs	diclofenac, ketoprofen, ketorolac
Steroids	beclomethasone, prednisone, triamcinolone

Patients may develop dysgeusia as a result of zinc deficiency.[22] While there is not sufficient evidence to recommend the routine use of zinc in all patients, zinc may play a role in hard to treat cases of dysgeusia.

MUCOSITIS

Chemotherapy-induced mucositis is one of the most problematic complications associated with antineoplastic therapy. Mucositis can become a dose limiting toxicity for many patients, and as a result they will not be able to receive the full course of their chemotherapy regimen. Chemotherapy induced mucositis can occur through two separate mechanisms.[34] Direct toxicity to the oral epithelium is perhaps the most obvious drug-induced cause. This usually occurs within five to ten days of medication administration. The other mechanism, indirect toxicity, can occur during the period of drug-induced neutropenia. During this time patients are prone to infections that can manifest as mucositis. The time course for indirect toxicity will depend upon the nadir of an individual chemotherapeutic agent. Culturing is critical at this point to differentiate chemotherapy-induced mucosal toxicity from mucosal neutropenic infectious complications caused by bacterial, fungal, or viral microorganisms. Mucosal herpes simplex virus infection can be an exception in relation to the time course development of mucositis. Such an occurrence can lead to significant misdiagnosis as direct mucositis and subsequent nontreatment of the infectious process. Whether a patient develops direct or indirect toxicity, infection must be recognized, properly diagnosed, and treated quickly and aggressively since systemic involvement can be life threatening.[14] The most frequently documented source of sepsis in the granulocytopenic cancer patient is the mouth.[14]

Chemotherapy responsible for mucositis includes alkylating agents, anthracyclines, antimetabolites, antineoplastic antibiotics, taxanes, and the vinca alkaloids. These agents cause mucosal ulceration by directly damaging the epithelium. Chemptherapeutic agents most commonly associated with mucositis include the following.

Chemotherapeutic Agents Commonly Associated with Mucositis[13,34-39]	
Class	*Examples*
Alkylating agents	busulfan, cyclophosphamide, procarbazine, thiotepa mechlorethamine (nitrogen mustard)
Anthracenes	daunorubicin, doxorubicin, epirubicin, mitoxantrone
Antimetabolites	cytarabine, floxuridine (FUDR), fluorouracil, hydroxyurea, methotrexate
Purine antagonists	6-mercaptopurine, 6-thioguanine
Antitumor antibiotics	bleomycin, dactinomycin, mitomycin, plicamycin
Plant alkaloids/Snythetic derivatives	etoposide, irinotecan, topotecan, vinblastine, vincristine, vinorelbine
Taxanes	docetaxel, paclitaxel

While the most common cause of drug-induced mucositis is cancer chemotherapy and radiotherapy, other agents have been implicated in drug-induced mucositis. The following list contains medications that have been implicated in mucositis.

Medications Associated with Mucositis[2,40,41]		
amitriptyline	amoxicillin	azathioprine
carbamazepine	ciprofloxacin	cyclobenzaprine
diclofenac	diflunisal	enalapril
erthyromycin	fluoxetine	ibuprofen
ketoprofen	ketorolac	lovastatin
nabumetone	naproxen	nicotine polacrilex
norfloxacin	nortriptyline	ofloxacin
penicillin	penicillamine	piroxicam
sulfasalazine	tetracycline	triazolam
trimetrexate	trimethoprim/sulfamethoxazole	

A number of these medications are commonly used in pain management and palliative care, such as carbamazepine, NSAIDs, and the tricyclic antidepressants. While the relative incidence of mucositis with these medications in the terminal population is not known, clinicians should be alert to mucosal injury that may result from use of these medications.

GENERAL CONSIDERATIONS

Chemotherapy-induced sequelae can include pancytopenia, nausea, mucositis, and infection.[8,42] To avoid such events, the patient should be advised of the importance of brushing with a soft toothbrush, keeping the oral mucosa moist and clean, and selecting and maintaining an appropriate diet during the period following cytotoxic therapy. The fear that brushing will increase the chances of oral complications has always been a concern for practitioners. The benefits of brushing outweigh the drawbacks. Even in healthy mouths, a certain degree of bacteremia can be associated with normal function, e.g., eating. However, any threat of persistent bacteremia in a compromised host is cause for concern. The benefits of controlling bacteremia-promoting plaque through appropriate hygiene (swishing fluids is a poor substitute for thorough oral care by brushing) far exceeds the drawback of a potential increase in oral complications. Careful oral care that includes brushing can keep chemotherapy-induced sequelae to a minimum, or even eradicate this problem.

Compliance with oral care procedures is essential to maintaining healthy mucosal tissues and the effectiveness of locally applied topical oral agents. Such topical medications should be nonirritating and non-dehydrating. Mouth rinses frequently are recommended as therapy for mucositis in both dentate and edentulous patients. Such rinses cleanse the mouth, hydrate the mucosa, and treat the mucositis. Any oral medications that contain alcohol, thymol, eugenol, or phenol, which are part of most commercial mouthwashes, should be avoided since they can irritate and desiccate inflamed, compromised xerostomic tissues.[43] Such rinses can lead to further compromise of the mucosa prolonging the healing of the oral wounds. Experience has shown that a diluted hydrogen peroxide solution (1:4, 3% hydrogen peroxide/water) adequately cleanses the tissues of debris, bacteria, and mucous.[7,9] This cleansing should be immediately followed by a mouth rinse of water. When oral lesions exist, rinsing with the hydrogen peroxide solution is only recommended to decrease wound contamination and colonization. The hydrogen peroxide rinse should not be used if there are any blood clots or bleeding since this would only encourage more bleeding.

Topical coating agents can be most effective in promoting mucosal wound healing and the sequence of delivery to the compromised oral soft tissues is important.[8,11] The tissue must be cleaned of mucoid debris before the application of the agents. Next, a troche or lozenge form of the medication should be taken, as it provides a longer and more constant application of the medicine to the tissue.[9] An oral liquid suspension can be used if the mouth is dry, even though the liquid will be in contact with the tissue and any organisms for only a limited time. All prostheses should be removed during the oral-mucosal treatment. If a mucosal coating agent is be used, it must be used last so as not to neutralize the effects of the topical antimicrobial agents. Thirty minutes should elapse between the applications of the agents. In providing the treatment described above, an oral care schedule for patients receiving chemotherapy can be very useful. Appropriate assessment and therapy depends on constant vigilance of oral mucosal wounds with appropriate cultures.

The use of topical anesthetic agents is discouraged because such agents are by nature irritants and they may suppress the gag-cough reflex leading to possible aspiration.

CONCLUSION

Patients near the end of life may be predisposed to problems of their oral mucosa. Oral mucositis is a common, dose-limiting, and potentially serious complication of both radiation therapy and chemotherapy. These therapies are nonspecific and interfere with the cellular homeostasis of both malignant and normal host cells. Currently, no evidence is available with regard to managing oral complications in the terminally ill. However, good information is available in the treatment for cure oncology literature which can serve as an initial reference point for those who care for dying patients. Future research must occur in this under-served population to give clinicians the opportunity to better care for these deserving patients.

SOME OPEN RESEARCH QUESTIONS

1. What are the actual prevalences of xerostomia and mucositis in palliative care patients?
2. How much does drug-induced dysgeusia impair eating and drinking in terminally ill patients?
3. What is the patient acceptance rate for available artificial saliva solutions?

TABLE 1. Treatment Options for Mucositis

Treatment	Uses	AWP per day[#]	Comments
intensive oral care	Prevention/Treatment	N/A	Should be standard treatment for all patients. Poses minimal risks to patients.
bland rinses (hydrogen peroxide and water)	Prevention/Treatment	N/A	Poses minimal risk to patients. May be useful in dehydrated patients.
cryotherapy	Can be used for painful lesions. May dry cavity. Probably a second line agent.	N/A	May be useful in preventing chemotherapy-induced oral pathology.
sucralfate (Carafate)	Cornerstone of effective pain management. Use in combination with other treatment modalities. (Refer to pain section)		Protects damaged mucosa. MUST rinse oral cavity prior to use. May dry oral cavity; encourage hydration and oral rinses.
vitamin E	Treatment		May promote healing of oral lesions.
viscous lidocaine	Treatment		
opioids (morphine)	Treatment		

Average Wholesale Price, 1999 (cost to pharmacy)

REFERENCES

1. Sweeney M, Bagg J. Oral care for hospice patients with advanced cancer. Dent Update. 1995;22:424-427.

2. Smith R, Burtner A. Oral side-effects of the most frequently prescribed drugs. Spec Care Dentist. 1994;14:96-102.

3. DeConno FR, Sbanotto A, Ventafridda V. Oral complications in patients with advanced cancer. J Pain Symptom Manage. 1989;4:20-30.

4. Wellman M, Jackson II K. Evidence-based management of mucositis: a systematic review of published trials. J Pharm Care Pain Symptom Control. 2000;8:In Press.

5. Greenberg M, Cohen S, McKitrick J, et al. The oral flora as a source of septicemia in patients with acute leukemia. Oral Surg Oral Med Oral Pathol. 1986; 315:1501-1505.

6. Bergman O. Oral infections and septicemia in immunocomprimised patients with hematologic malignancies. J Clin Microbiol. 1988;26:2105-2109.

7. Toth B, Martin J, Fleming T. Oral complications associated with cancer therapy: An M.D. Anderson Cancer Center experience. J Clin Periodontol. 1990;17:508-515.

8. Toth B, Frame R. Dental oncology: The management of disease and treatment-related oral/dental complications associated with chemotherapy. Curr Probl Cancer. 1983;7:7-35.

9. Toth B, Martin J, Fleming T. Oral and dental care associated with cancer therapy. Cancer Bull. 1991;43:397-402.

10. Lindquist S, Hickey A, Drane J. Effects of oral hygiene on stomatitis in patients receiving cancer chemotherapy. J Prosthet Dent. 1978;40:312-314.

11. King G, Toth B, Fleming T. Oral dental care of the cancer patient. Texas Dent J. 1988;105:10-11.

12. Sonis S, Clark J. Prevention and management of oral mucositis induced by antineoplastic therapy. Oncology. 1991;5:11-18.

13. Parulekar W, Mackenzie R, Bjarnason G, Jordan R. Scoring oral mucositis. Oral Oncology. 1998;34:63-71.

14. Sonis S, Fazio R, Fang L. Principles and practice of oral medicine Philadelphia, PA: WB Saunders; 1984:492-542.

15. Chambers M, Toth B, Martin J, Fleming T, Lemon J. Oral and dental management of the cancer patient: prevention and treatment of complications. Support Care Cancer. 1995;3:168-175.

16. Marciani R, Ownby H. Osteoradionecrosis of the jaws. J Oral Maxillofac Surg. 1986;4:218-223.

17. Epstein J, Giuseppe R, Wong F, et al. Osteoradionecrosis: Study of the relationship of dental extractions in patients receiving radiotherapy. Head Neck Surg. 1987;10:48-54.

18. Schweiger J. Oral complications following radiation therapy: a five-year retrospective report. J Prosthet Dent. 19887;58:778-782.

19. Fleming T. Oral tissue changes of radiation-oncology and their management. Dent Clin North Am. 1990;34:233-237.

20. Liu R, Fleming T, Toth B, et al. Salivary flow rates in patients with head and neck cancer 0.5 to 25 years after radiotherapy. Oral Surg Oral Med Oral Pathol. 1990;70:724-729.

21. Chambers M. Xerostomia and its role in mucositis: Complications and management. Ninth International MASCC Symposium (abstract). Support Care Cancer. 1997;5:149.

22. Ventafridda V, Ripamonte C, Sbanotto A, De Conno F. Mouth care. In: Doyle D, Hanks G, MacDonald N, eds. Oxford Textbook of Palliative Medicine. 2nd ed. Oxford: Oxford University Press; 1998:691-707.

23. Berger A, Kilroy T. Oral complications of cancer therapy. In: Berger A, Portenoy R, Weissman D, eds. Principles and Practices of Supportive Oncology. Philadelphia: Lippincott-Raven; 1998:223-236.

24. Rothwell B. Prevention and treatment of the orofacial complications of radiotherapy. JADA. 1987;114:316-322.

25. Felder R, Millar S. Dental care of the polymedication patient. Dent Clin North Am. 1994;38:525-536.

26. Carl W. Oral complications of local and systemic cancer treatment. Curr Opin Oncol. 1995;7:320-324.

27. Sreebny L, Schwartz S. A reference guide to drugs and dry mouth–2nd edition. Gerodontology. 1997;14:33-47.

28. Navazesh M. Xerostomia in the aged. Dent Clin North Am. 1989;33:75-80.

29. Terezhalmy G. Adverse drug effects. Dent Clin North Am. 1994;38:769-783.

30. Paunovich E, Sadowsky J, Carter P. The most frequently prescribed medications in the elderly and their impact on dental treatment. Dent Clin North Am. 1997;41:699-726.

31. Fox P. Management of dry mouth. Dent Clin North Am. 1997;41:863-874.

32. Mandel I. The role of saliva in maintaining oral homeostasis. J Am Dent Assoc. 1989;119:298-303.

33. Keene H, Fleming T. Prevalence of caries-associated microflora after radiotherapy in patients with cancer of the head and neck. Oral Surg Oral Med Oral Pathol. 1987;64:421-426.

34. Verdi C. Cancer therapy and oral mucositis–An appraisal of drug prophylaxis. Drug Safety. 1993;9:185-195.

35. Oral Complications of Cancer Therapies: Diagnosis P, and Treatment. NIH Consens Statement Online. 1989 Apr 17-19;7:1-11.

36. Wilkes J. Prevention and treatment of oral mucositis following cancer chemotherapy. Semin Oncol. 1998;25:538-551.

37. Tipton J, Skeel R. Management of acute side effects of cancer chemotherapy. In: Skeel R, Lachant N, eds. Handbook of Cancer Chemotherapy, 4th ed. Boston: Little, Brown, and Company; 1995:573-589.

38. National Cancer Institute. Oral complications of cancer and cancer therapy. http://cancernet.nci.nih.gov/clinpdq/supportive/Oralcomplications_of_cancer_and_ cancer _therapy.Physician.html 1998.

39. Carnel S, Blakeslee D, Oswald S, Barnes M. Treatment of radiation and chemotherapy-induced stomatitis. Otolaryngol Head Neck Surg. 1990;102:326-330.

40. Balmer C, Wells AV. Basic principles of cancer treatment and cancer chemotherapy. In Pharmacotherapy, 3rd edition, Dipiro J. Talbert R, Yee G, et al., editors, Stamford CT. Appleton and Lange, 1997.

41. Knoben JE, Anderson PO. Handbook of Clinical Drug Data, 8 ed. Stamford, CT: Appleton and Lange; 1997.

42. King G, Lemon J, Martin J. Multidisciplinary teamwork in the treatment and rehabilitation of the head and neck cancer patient. Texas Dent J. 1992;109:9-12.

43. Kaminski S, Gillette W, O'Leary T. Sodium absorption associated with oral hygiene procedures. JADA. 1987;114:644-646.

Nausea and Vomiting in Palliative Care

Linda S. Tyler

SUMMARY. Nausea and vomiting occur commonly in palliative care patients and these symptoms are usually manageable. Identification of the cause(s) is important in planning therapy. Common causes, general treatment measures and drug therapy are summarized. Evaluation instruments that have been used to assess these symptoms are described. Some open research questions are listed. A treatment algorithm, evidence tables and drug therapy tables are which include drug costs are presented. *[Article copies available for a fee from The Haworth Document Delivery Service: 1-800-342-9678. E-mail address: getinfo@haworthpressinc. com <Website: http://www.haworthpressinc.com>]*

KEYWORDS. Nausea, vomiting, gastric, irritation, distention, fecal impaction, emotions, pain, fear, meningitis, intracranial pressure, palliative care, terminal care, dying, supportive care, drug therapy, non-pharmacological therapy, etiology, evidence, costs, algorithm, dopamine antagonists, antimuscarinic, antihistamines, anticholinergic, serotonin receptor antagonists, prokinetic agents, metoclopramide, cisapride, cannabinoids, corticosteroids, steroids, prednisone, dexamethasone, antianxiety, octreotide, phenothiazines, butyrophenones, promethazine, methotrimeprazine, haloperidol, ondansetron, meclizine, cyclizine, dimenhydrinate, lorazepam, alprazolam

---

Linda S. Tyler, PharmD, is Professor, College of Pharmacy; and Manager, Drug Information Service, Department of Pharmacy Services, University Hospitals and Clinics; University of Utah Health Sciences Center, Salt Lake City, UT.

Address correspondence to: Arthur G. Lipman, PharmD, College of Pharmacy and Pain Management Center, 30 S 2000 E RM 258, University of Utah Health Sciences Center, Salt Lake City, UT 84112-5820 (E-mail: alipman@pharm.utah.edu).

[Haworth co-indexing entry note]: "Nausea and Vomiting in Palliative Care." Tyler, Linda S. Co-published simultaneously in *Journal of Pharmaceutical Care in Pain & Symptom Control* (Pharmaceutical Products Press, an imprint of The Haworth Press, Inc.) Vol. 8, No. 1, 2000, pp. 163-181; and: *Evidence Based Symptom Control in Palliative Care: Systematic Reviews and Validated Clinical Practice Guidelines for 15 Common Problems in Patients with Life Limiting Disease* (ed: Arthur G. Lipman, Kenneth C. Jackson II, and Linda S. Tyler) Pharmaceutical Products Press, an imprint of The Haworth Press, Inc., 2000, pp. 163-181. Single or multiple copies of this article are available for a fee from The Haworth Document Delivery Service [1-800-342-9678, 9:00 a.m. - 5:00 p.m. (EST). E-mail address: getinfo@haworthpressinc. com].

163

Algorithm for Managing Nausea and Vomiting in Palliative Care

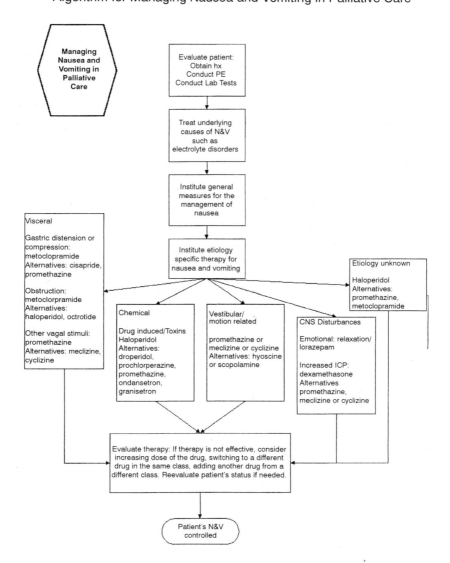

Nausea and vomiting are common, troublesome, multifactorial symptoms in terminally ill patients. Reuben and Mor[1] estimated that 62% of terminally ill patients developed nausea and vomiting, with 40% having symptoms in the last 6 weeks of life. However, little evidence is available that has evaluated the most effective way to manage these symptoms. Much of the literature on managing severe nausea and vomiting is based on patients who have received chemotherapy. Because chemotherapy-induced nausea and vomiting differs both in mechanism and pathophysiology from nausea and vomiting due directly to advanced disease, those findings may not be applicable in terminal care. Of the evidence available on terminally ill patients, most are descriptive case reports or case series. (Table 1)

Several authors have reviewed this topic.[2-8] Lichter[3,4] described a protocol used in 100 terminally ill patients. Control of symptoms was achieved in 70% of patients within 24 hours, and 93% within 48 hours. Lichter's approach is to assess the causes of nausea and vomiting and to select receptor-specific antiemetic agents. The drug therapy choices in this protocol were based on neurotransmitter receptor binding studies conducted by Ison[9] and Peroutka.[10] Basing drug therapy on probable receptors provides a systematic process for evaluating and managing patients' symptoms. The following steps are useful in evaluating patients and determining the treatment options.

EVALUATE THE ETIOLOGY

Nausea and vomiting may be due to many factors. There are four general mechanisms involved in the pathophysiology of nausea and vomiting:

- visceral or gastrointestinal tract disorders
- chemical triggers
- central nervous system disturbances
- vestibular disturbances.

Nausea also may be triggered by a bad taste in mouth, specific foods, odors, and pain. Several assessment tools may help assess probable cause(s) and optimal treatment(s) for nausea and vomiting.

TABLE 1. Drug Therapy for Managing Nausea and Vomiting in Palliative Care–Evidence Tables

Reference	Study Design	n	Intervention	Results	Level of Evidence	Comments
Ondansetron (Zofran)						
Marsden (1993)[13] {editorial}	Descriptive	3	Ondansetron was used by 3 terminally ill patients. (Dose listed as 8 mg q8h for one of the patients.) All had failed previous antiemetic therapy.	"Dramatic" improvement within 24 hours in 2 patients and several days in the other. Allowed two patients to return home for her last days. Controlled nausea in another patient until she developed a bowel obstruction.	V	
Andrews (1995) {editorial}	Descriptive n of 1 trial	2	Oral ondansetron 8 mg twice daily in 2 terminal uremia patients who had failed metoclopramide therapy. (Report also describes results in 2 nonterminal dialysis patients.)	Patients responded within 24 hours. One patient withdrawn from therapy and symptoms returned; therapy was reinstituted. The other patient also noted improvement in pruritus symptoms.	V	
Cole (1994)	Descriptive	1	Ondansetron 8 mg over 8 hours in an advanced cancer patient. Haloperidol 1.5 mg HS also was used. Patient failed metoclopramide, haloperidol, promethazine, hyoscine, meclizine)	With ondansetron, patient was able to remain free of nausea for 10 weeks prior to her death. Occasional vomiting did occur in the two weeks before she died.	V	
Pereira (1996)	Descriptive	1	Ondansetron 8 mg q12h in a patient with advanced cancer. Patient failed previous therapy including metoclopramide, dexamethasone, chlorpromazine, lorazepam dimenhydrinate.	Patient responded to therapy within 24 hours. Other therapies were discontinued	V	
Octreotide (Sandostatin) [in patients with bowel obstruction who were not surgical candidates]						
Khoo (1992)[17] {editorial}	Descriptive n of 1 trial	5	octreotide 100 mcg, followed by 300 mcg/ continuous infusion in 4 patients; 50 mcg tid in the other.	Vomiting ceased within 1 hour of initiating therapy in all patients. Two patients had therapy stopped with return of symptoms within 12 hours; symptoms resolved on restarting the drug.	V	Unclear if these patients were included in subsequent report, but based on patient detail, probably not.
Mercadante (1993)[18]	Descriptive	1 4	Octreotide 300-600 mcg by SQ bolus or continuous infusion in terminally ill cancer patients who had failed other therapy.	12 patients experienced relief of symptoms	V	Octreotide was administered until at least one day before death.

Study	Type		Description	Level	Comments
Khoo (1994)[19] Riley (1994)[20]	Descriptive	2 4	Octreotide 50 mcg tid SQ. Dose was increased by 50 mcg based on response. (Used SQ for first two patients then used continuous SQ infusion for the remainder.) Once response achieved, the dose was decreased ~150 mcg/d in most patients. These terminally ill patients had failed to respond to other antiemetic therapies.	V	Continuous infusion was preferred to prevent multiple injections for patients. Same data reported in both publications. Khoo, et al., includes more details on methodology.
Mangili (1996)[21]	Descriptive	1 3	Octreotide 300-600 mcg/d SQ or by continuous infusion in patients with advanced ovarian cancer who had failed therapy with haloperidol and metoclopramide.	V	All patients responded with complete control of vomiting. NG tube was removed in all patients. 8 patients were discharged home. One patient developed small bowel necrosis above the obstruction.
Nabilone (no longer available in the U.S.)					
Flynn (1992)[22]	Descriptive	1	Nabilone 2 mg bid was reduced after 1 week to 1 mg bid in an HIV-positive patient who had failed scopolamine, dimenhydrinate, and prochlorperazine.	V	Controlled nausea until patient died.
Green (1989)[23] (editorial)	Descriptive	1	Nabilone 1 mg bid in a terminally ill, HIV-positive patient. Patient had failed other therapy including prochlorperazine, cyclizine, domperidone, and metoclopramide.	V	"Complete cessation" of nausea and vomiting.
Phenothiazines/Butyrophenones					
Baines (1985)	Descriptive	4 0	Patients had intestinal obstruction, 37 had previous surgery for obstruction. methotrimeprazine (no longer available in the U.S.) 50-150 mg/d constant infusion; haloperidol 5-10 mg/24 hours PO or parenteral; cyclizine 150 mg/d.	V	Prior to therapy, 12 patients reported severe vomiting and 21 moderate. After treatment, 4 reported severe symptoms 29 had mild symptoms, and 5 had no symptoms.	Metoclopramide and domperidone not effective and worsened colic. Report unclear on how the therapies were used; outcomes not discussed.

Key to Level of Evidence classification:

Level I   Randomized trials with low false-positive (alpha) and low false-negative (beta errors); high power
Level II   Randomized trials with high false-positive (alpha) and/or high false-negative (beta errors); low power
Level III Non-randomized concurrent cohort comparisons between contemporaneous patients who did and did not receive a given intervention
Level IV   Non-randomized historical cohort comparisons between current patients who did receive the intervention and patients (from the same institution or from the literature) who did not
Level V   Case series without control subjects

N of 1 studies are case reports in which an individual patient received therapy which subsequently was stopped and later restarted (challenge, dechallenge, rechallenge)

STEPS IN DEFINING OPTIMAL THERAPY

Obtain a patient history. Information should be obtained from the patient concerning timing, frequency and characteristics of symptoms. Patients should be asked if any particular events trigger their symptoms, in particular if any drugs, foods, or situations change their symptoms.

Conduct a patient physical examination with particular attention to the oral, abdominal, rectal, and neurological exam. Conduct laboratory tests to determine if the patient has electrolyte, fluid, or chemical imbalances associated with nausea and vomiting, i.e., hypercalcemia, hyponatremia, uremia, hypovolemia. These steps should help the clinician to identify the potential causes of the patient's nausea.

Treat Underlying Causes of Nausea and Vomiting

Nausea and vomiting often are caused by other disorders for which clinicians should initiate indicated medical or surgical management. Electrolyte disorders should be corrected if possible. Patients with obstructed bowel may be surgical candidates if their life expectancy and probability of gaining sufficient quality of life favor surgery. Most terminally ill patients are not surgical candidates.

Institute General Treatment Management Measures for Nausea

For many patients, the following measures may help decrease their symptoms. Any of the following that are appropriate for the patient should be instituted.[8] Provide small, frequent meals, composed of foods chosen by the patient. Patient should avoid foods that are disagreeable or have disagreeable odors. Fatty and fried foods should be avoided.

Advanced disease patients often have decreased taste (hypogeusia). When that occurs, patients often prefer different foods than they liked previously.

Advanced disease patients sometimes experience altered taste (dysgeusia) which can cause previously favored foods to be disagreeable. This may occur with sweet tasting foods such as candies and cherry flavored syrups, and urea containing foods such as meat. In such cases, bland flavors often are more acceptable.

POTENTIALLY USEFUL STRATEGIES

- Provide liquids frequently.
- Provide a quiet, relaxing, pleasant atmosphere for the patient.
- Provide companionship for meals.
- Teach the patient relaxation techniques.
- Encourage the patient to get enough rest.
- Have the patient take medications after meals if possible, except for antiemetic therapy.
- Have the patient try an alcoholic beverage before meals if desired.
- Wine based aperitifs are often better tolerated than whiskey.
- Keep the patient's mouth clean and moist.
- Foul taste in the mouth may make symptoms worse.
- Remove foul odors.
- Administer a topical antifungal (e.g., nystatin) if patient has thrush.
- Use hydration (water bottle) in an oxygen line.
- Institute etiology-specific therapy for nausea and vomiting.

Probable etiology of the nausea and vomiting should be the basis of therapy selected for the patient. While few data are available, drug therapy may be recommended based on its pharmacologic properties. Table 2 outlines the therapy choices based on etiology. The following drug classes frequently are used in the management of nausea and vomiting.

Dopamine Antagonists

Dopamine receptors are involved in nausea and vomiting especially when these symptoms are caused by gastric stasis and chemically-induced causes. Phenothiazines and butyrophenones are the two major pharmacological classes used as dopamine antagonists. Prochlorperazine is available as oral tablets, oral liquid, rectal suppositories and parenteral dosage forms. The long acting (12 hour) capsules offer little advantage over less expensive oral dosage forms because the oral tablets and liquids routinely provide 6 and often 8 hours of relief. Chlorpromazine is an acceptable alternative when more sedation is wanted. Fluphenazine is more potent than prochlorperazine, but usually is too sedating to be useful. Prochlorperazine is less sedating than

TABLE 2. Selecting Therapy for Nausea and Vomiting Based on Etiology

Visceral disturbances
Receptors involved: **Vagal and sympathetic afferents, vomiting center** H_1 = Histamine, M = Muscarinic cholinergic, $5HT_3$ = Serotonin group 3
For gastric statis also: D_2 = Dopamine D_2, $5HT_4$ = Serotonin Group 4

Etiology	Initial Therapy of Choice	Alternative Therapies	AWP per Day of Therapy#	Comments
Gastric irritation drugs	Discontinue drug if possible; give drugs with food or an antacid 30 mL po qid	Add a histamine₂ antagonist: (select least expensive) cimetidine 300 mg po qid famotidine 20 mg po bid ranitidine 150 mg po bid nizatidine 150 mg po bid Add a cytoprotective agent: sucralfate 1 g PO or misoprostol 20 mcg PO qid	$0.050 $0.99 $3.08 $1.91 $3.16 $2.94 $2.82	Nausea and vomiting from this cause is not treated with antiemetic agents.
Gastric Distension Statis Statis due to opioids Excess food intake	metoclopramide 10-20 mg po q6h	cisapride 10 mg PO qid promethazine 25-50 mg PO q6h metoclopramide 10-20 mg IV q6h promethazine 50-100 ng PR q6h	$0.08-0.15 $2.51 $0.05-0.19 $4.56-9.12 $12.16-24.32	Metoclopramide has been used by continuous SQ infusion[3,5]
Intestinal obstruction	metoclopramide 10-20 mg po q6h	haloperidol 0.5-2 mg PO q6h metoclopramide 10-20 mg IV q6h haloperidol 0.5-2 mg IM q6h octreotide 150 mcg-600 mcg SQ constant infusion or in 3 divided doses	$0.08-0.15 $0.08 $4.46-9.12 $1.18-4.73 $7.08-28.32	Metoclopramide and haloperidol have been used by continuous SQ infusion[3,5]
Gastric compression	metoclopramide (Reglan) 10 mg po q6h	cisapride 10 mg PO qid metoclopramide 10-20 mg IV q6h	$0.08-0.15 $2.51 $4.46-9.12	
Other vagal afferent stimuli Abdominal cancer Stomach cancer External pressure Constipation Genitourinary distension Biliary distension Peritoneal inflammation Cardiac pain	promethazine (Phenrgan) 25-50 mg po q6h (frequency may be increaesed to q4h if desired)	meclizine 25-50 mg po qid cyclizine 50 mg po q6h promethazine 25-50 mg IM q6h promethazine 50-100 mg PR q6h	$0.05-0.19 $0.12-0.24 $2.07-2.56 $12.16-24.32	Meclizine and cyclizine available as OTC products.

Chemical causes Receptors involved: Chemoreceptor trigger zone, D_2 = Dopamine 2 receptor, $5HT_3$ = Serotonin group 3, vomiting center, H_1 = Histamine, M = Muscarinic cholinergic

Cause	Management	Drug / Dose	Cost	Notes
Drugs	Discontinue if possible	haloperidol 0.5-2 mg PO q6h	$0.08	Haloperidol has been used by continuous SQ infusion
		0.5-2 mg IM q6h	$1.18-4.76	
		(Dosing interval may be to q4h) OR		
		prochlorperazine 5-10 mg PO q6h		
		spansules 10-20 mg PO q12h	$1.36-3.06	
		25 mg PR q6h	$2.12-4.24	
		5-10 mg IM q6h		
		(Dosing frequency may be to q4h though not on the spansules)	$7.71 $11.95-35.85	
		ADD		
		promethazine 25-50 mg PO q6h	$0.10-0.19h	
		promethazine 25-50 mg IM q6h	$2.07-2.56	
		promethazine 50-100 mg PR q6h	$12.16-24.32	
		(Dosing frequency may be to q4h)		
		CHANGE TO:		
		ondansetron 8 mg PO q8h	$56.10	
		ondansetron 8 mg IV q8h	$279.60	
		OR		
		granisetron 1 mg PO bid	$78.75	
		granisetron 1 mg IV bid	$332.00	
Toxins Tumor-produced peptides Infection Radiotherapy Abnormal cancer metabolites	haloperidol (Haldol) 0.5-2 mg po q6h 0.5-2 mg IM q6h (Dosing frequency may be increased to q4h)	droperidol 1-2 mg SQ q4h CHANGE TO:	$0.08	
		ondansetron 8 mg po q8h	$1.18-4.73	
		ondansetron 8 mg IV q8h	$3.72-7.44	
		OR	$56.10	
		granisetron 1 mg po bid	$279.60	
		granisetron 1 mg IV bid	$78.75	
			$332.00	
Biochemical Disorders Uremia Hypercalcemia SIADH Volume depletion	Manage underlying cause Hypercalcemia dexamethasone or prednisone			

TABLE 2 (continued)

Etiology	Initial Therapy of Choice	Alternative Therapies	AWP per Day of Therapy#	Comments
Vestibular disturbances (Motion Related nausea)				
Receptors involved: Vestibular nuclei, M = Muscarinic cholinergic, H$_1$ = Histamine, vomiting center, H$_1$ = Histamine, 5HT$_3$ = Serotonin group 3				
Diagnostic Clues: Nausea and vomiting most likely due to vestibular causes if patient experiences increased symptoms when: Walking, bending over then standing up, signs and symptoms of middle ear infection				
Drugs Aspirin Opioids	Discontinue drug if possible	Choose one of the following: promethazine 25-50 mg po q6h (frequency may be increased to q4h if desired) meclizine 25-50 mg po qid cyclizine 50 mg po q6h promethazine 25-50 mg IM q6h promethazine 50-100 mg PR q6h ADD EITHER: Hyoscine 0.125-0.25 mg q4h (PO, sublingual or chewable) (elixir 0.125 mg/5 mL) sustained release 0.375 mg capsules 1-2 q12h; OR scopolamine 0.4-0.6 mg SQ OR IM q6-8h	$0.05-0.19 $0.12-0.24 $2.07-2.56 $12.16-24.32 $0.45-0.90 $0.50-1.00 $1.00-2.00 $3.60-4.80	Scopolamine patches not currently available in the United States.
Local tumors Brain tumors Acoustic neuroma Bone metastases at base of skull Motion sickness Meniere disease Labyrinthitis	promethazine (Phenergan) 25-50 mg po q6h (frequency may be increased to q4h if desired)	Choose one of the following: meclizine 25-50 mg PO qid cyclizine 50 mg PO q6h promethazine 25-50 mg IM q6h promethazine 50-100 mg PR q6h ADD EITHER: Hyoscine 0.125-0.25 mg q4h (po, sublingual or chewable) (elixir 0.125 mg/5 mL) sustained release 0.375 mg capsules 1-2 q12h OR scopolamine 0.4-0.6 mg SQ or IM q6-8h	$0.05-0.19 $0.12-0.24 $2.07-2.56 $12.16-24.32 $0.45-0.90 $0.50-1.00 $1.00-2.00 $3.60-4.80	

172

Central Nervous System Disturbances
Receptors involved: Vomiting center, H_1 = Histamine; M = Muscarinic cholinergic; $5HT_3$ = Serotonin group 3.
For CNS cancer and raised ICP also: H_2 = Histamine 1
Diagnostic Clues: Often accompanied by other neurologic signs and symptoms, or mental status problems.

Emotional factors Pain Fear	Try relaxation techniques	Antianxiety agents lorazepam 1-2 mg po q6h 1-2 mg IV q6h	$0.67-0.74 $10.76-21.52	Oral lorazepam may be given sublingually.
CNS cancer				
Raised intracrania pressure Inflammation secondary to radiotherapy	dexamethasone (Decadron) 1-4 mg po q6-8h (elixir) 1-4 mg IV q6-12 h	ADD promethazine 25-50 mg PO q6h increase to q4h if needed meclizine 25-50 mg PO qid cyclizine 50 mg PO q6h promethazine 25-50 mg IM q6h promethazine 50-100 mg PR q6h	$1.75-2.33 $1.90-7.63 $0.45-1.79 $0.05-0.19 $0.12-0.24 $2.07-2.56 $12.16-24.32	
Meningitis Chemical, Infectious Carcinomatous	Treat cause or meningitis: If chemical d/c drug Antibiotic therapy			
Etiology Unknown				
	haloperidol (Haldol) 0.5-2 mg po q6h 0.5-2 mg IM q6h (Dosing frequency may be increased to q4h)	Add an antihistamine: promethazine 25-50 mg po q6h promethazine 25-50 mg IM q6h promethazine 50-100 mg PR q6h (Dosing frequency may be increased to q4h) ADD: metoclopramide 10-20 mg po q6h 10-20 mg IV q6h In selected patients: dronabinol 2.5 mg bid-tid	$0.08 $1.18-4.73 $0.05-0.19 $2.07-2.56 $12.16-24.32 $0.08-0.15 $4.56-9.12 $5.78-8.67	Haloperidol and metoclopramide have been used by continuous SQ infusion[3,5]

Average Wholesale Price, 1999 (cost to pharmacy)

most other phenothiazines. Haloperidol is a potent, effective antiemetic.[9] Droperidol also is effective, but is more sedating than haloperidol.

Metoclopramide has dopamine antagonist action, especially at high doses. It is an antiemetic of choice when both dopamine antagonism and gastrokinesis (see below) are desired.

Histamine₁/Muscarinic (Cholinergic, Parasympathetic) Receptor Blockers

The histamine$_1$ receptor is involved in nausea caused by CNS cancer, elevated intracranial pressure (ICP), vestibular mechanisms (motion sickness), and stimulation of the medullary vomiting center. Cyclizine, meclizine, promethazine, and hydroxyzine are useful for nausea associated with this receptor. Diphenhydramine is less potent. Cyclizine and meclizine are first line drugs for this type of nausea because they have fewer side effects than the other agents and are inexpensive, nonprescription medications. Promethazine may causes excessive sedation.

Muscarinic (cholinergic, parasympathetic) receptors are involved in nausea and vomiting caused by vestibular mechanisms and at the medullary vomiting center. Antihistamines (histamine$_1$ receptor blockers) produce anticholinergic effects. The specific mechanism by which these drugs act as antiemetics (antihistamine or anticholinergic *per se*) is not clear. Hyoscine and scopolamine are potent antimuscarinic drugs. These drugs cause more marked anticholinergic side effects than the antihistamines listed above. Promethazine also demonstrates some antimuscarinic activity. The potent antimuscarinic agents usually should be reserved for use in motion-exacerbated nausea which does not respond to the recommended antihistamines.

Serotonin Receptor Antagonists

The serotonin (5-HT$_3$) receptor is involved in nausea and vomiting caused by the chemoreceptor trigger zone and the central vomiting center. Ondansetron, granisetron and dolasetron are available in the United States. These drugs have revolutionized the management of chemotherapy-induced nausea and vomiting. Little information is available on the use of 5HT$_3$ blockers in other types of nausea and vomiting. Some clinicians advocate use of these drugs in intractable nausea and vomiting based on clinical experience. These very expensive agents should be reserved for use after trying other antiemetics.

Prokinetic Agents

Metoclopramide blocks the serotonin 5-HT$_4$ receptors, increasing gastric motility above the jejunum. These receptors are involved in nausea and vomiting caused by visceral distention. It is preferred by many because it has fewer CNS effects. Metoclopramide also blocks dopamine receptors at regular doses and serotonin 5-HT$_3$ receptors at higher doses.

Cisapride is a prokinetic drug which may also reduce afferent activity in the vagal nerve and act on acetylcholine receptors in the myenteric plexis. Its prokinetic effect is throughout the GI tract. Because it lacks dopamine activity, it is not as useful as metoclopramide as an antiemetic.

Cannabinoids

While many advocate the use of cannabinoids to treat nausea and vomiting, few data are available. Dronabinol is available orally. Nabilone (no longer available in the U.S.) has been used in other countries. Some authors recommend smoking marijuana.[11,12] The mechanism and the role of marijuana in therapy in palliative care are unclear. Endogenous cannabinoid receptors have been identified and cloned. These receptors play a not yet fully defined role in the effects of these drugs.

Corticosteroids

The role of corticosteroids in the management of nausea and vomiting is unclear. These drugs may inhibit the synthesis of prostaglandins which may play a role in vomiting. They are used when CNS tumor is present to decrease the inflammation and intracranial pressure. Dexamethasone is the preferred agent because it has lower mineralocorticoid (sodium retaining) properties than most other glucocorticoids. Prednisone (orally) and methylprednisolone (parenterally) are alternatives. While some have advocated steroids in nausea and vomiting of non-specific causes, there is not evidence to support such use. Steroids may cause gastric irritation which could exacerbate nausea in some patients.

Antianxiety Agents

Lorazepam and alprazolam have been used extensively in palliative care. Lorazepam has been used more extensively in preventing nausea due to chemotherapy, especially if anticipatory nausea and vomiting were potential issues. Psychological desensitization is more effective than relaxation therapy or medications to treat anticipatory vomiting.

Octreotide

Surgery is the treatment of choice for bowel obstruction, but surgery is not always appropriate or possible in terminally ill patients. Bowel obstruction is common in persons with advanced cancer and some other palliative care patients. Octreotide is a somatostatin analogue that has been highly effective in stopping vomiting of patients with bowel obstruction by decreasing intestinal secretions. Infusions of 300 mcg of octreotide stopped intractable vomiting in some terminally ill patients within an hour. It is doubtful if the drug would be effective at doses above 600 mcg per day.

CONCLUSION

If initial therapy is not effective, the clinician should evaluate the patient's response and consider the following: increase the dose of the agent selected, try a different drug from the same class–especially if a particular side effect is an issue, add an additional agent from another drug class and reevaluate the cause(s) of the symptoms and select another agent accordingly.

EVALUATION OF NAUSEA AND VOMITING

One of the biggest problems in evaluating literature on nausea and vomiting is the lack of standardized methods and instruments to evaluate this in patients. Most of the tools have been used to assess nausea and vomiting due to chemotherapy. Some tools are used to determine the characteristics of the nausea and vomiting symptoms, while others focus on the effect of these symptoms on activities of daily living or quality of life. The following summarizes some of the tools and information available on this topic.

Palliative Care

Only two references specifically address nausea and vomiting in a patient population receiving palliative care.

1. Bruera E, Kuehn N, Miller MJ, et al. The Edmonton Symptom Assessment System (ESAS): a simple method for the assessment of palliative care patients. J Palliative Care 1991;7(2):6-9.[25]

This paper describes a 9 question tool to assess patients' symptoms using a VAS score. Symptoms assessed included pain, activity, nausea, depression, anxiety, drowsiness, appetite, sense of well being and shortness of breath.

2. Fainsinger R, Miller MJ, Bruera E, et al. Symptom control during the last week of life on a palliative care unit. J Palliative Care 1991; 7(1):5-11.[26]

The authors describe the use of ESAS twice daily to assess symptoms in 100 patients admitted to a palliative care unit for 6 or more days prior to death.

Chemotherapy-Induced Nausea and Vomiting

The majority of the literature available on evaluating nausea and vomiting are conducted in patients with nausea and vomiting related to chemotherapy. While several tools have been used, the FLIE and MANE are the ones most commonly used at this point.

3. Lindley CM, Hirsch JD, O'Neill CV et al. Quality of life consequences of chemotherapy-induced emesis. Quality Life Research 1992; 1:331-340.[27]

This article describes the use of the Functional Living Index–Emesis (FLIE) tool. This instrument is an 18 question, VAS from 1-7, that assesses the effect of nausea and vomiting on quality of life (QOL) indicators.

4. Morrow GR. A patient report measure for the quantification of chemotherapy induced nausea and emesis: Psychometric properties of the Morrow assessment of nausea and emesis (MANE). Br J Cancer 1992;19:S72-S74.[28]

The 5 question tool asks patients if they have experienced nausea or vomiting after chemotherapy and to assess the extent (6 point ordinal scale) of symptoms and when the symptoms were the worse.

5. Morrow GR. The assessment of nausea and vomiting: Past problems, current issues, and suggestions for future research. Cancer 1984;53:2267-2278.[29]

Though dated, this provides a good review of the problems and methods used to assess nausea and vomiting. This article presents the background for the MANE as well as the preliminary reliability and validity assessments with this instrument.

6. Bliss JM, Robertson B, Selby PJ. The impact of nausea and vomiting upon quality of life measures. Br J Cancer 1992; 19:S14-S23.[30]

This paper reviews tools used to assess QOL in cancer patients. In addition to the FLIE and MANE, the following tools were described to assess QOL in cancer patients. (Several tools were discussed; only the ones that assessed nausea and vomiting are included.)

The Rotterdam symptom checklist: 30 questions asking if patients have experienced a variety of symptoms, rated on a 4 point ordinal scale, plus 8 questions related to ability to perform activities of daily living, evaluated on a 4 point ordinal scale.

The EORTC Core Quality of Life Questionnaire: This includes 7 questions related to activities of daily living (yes/no), and 21 questions asking patients if they have experienced symptoms (rated on a 4 point ordinal scale). Two final questions ask patients how they have felt overall (rated on a 7 point ordinal scale).

The paper then goes on to assess if nausea and vomiting were independent predictors of QOL in patients receiving chemotherapy. The authors concluded that they were not.

7. Melzack R, Rosberger Z, Hollingsworth ML, et al. New approaches to measuring nausea. Can Med Assoc J 1985;133: 755-58.[31]

These researchers describe a 3 question instrument. The first question asks patients to check the descriptors that describe their symptoms. The second asks for an overall nausea index (ONI) (0-5 point ordinal scale). The third question is a VAS scale asking patients to mark extent of nausea.

8. Del Favero AD, Roila F, Basurto C, et al. Assessment of nausea. Eur J Clin Pharmacol 1990;38:115-120.[32]

The authors compared the results of using single question 4 point ordinal scale, versus a VAS question, versus a continuous chromatic analogue scale. These measures correlated with each other.

SOME OPEN RESEARCH QUESTIONS

1. What is the antihistamine drug of choice for managing nausea and vomiting?
2. What distinguishes when one agent in this class is preferred to another?
3. When are corticosteroids indicated? Is there a preference between agents?
4. When are cannabinoids recommended? Do they have a role in palliative care?
5. What is the role of granisetron and ondansetron in the management of nausea and vomiting in palliative care?
6. When is a change in therapy or the initiation of combination therapy indicated?
7. How do potential adverse effects influence your choice of therapy?
8. When is continuous subcutaneous infusion indicated?

REFERENCES

1. Reuben DB, Mor VM. Nausea and vomiting in terminal cancer patients. Arch Intern Med 1986; 146:2021-2023.

2. Rousseau P. Antiemetic therapy in adults with terminal disease: A brief review. Am J Hospice Palliat Care 1995; Jan/Feb:12-18.

3. Lichter I. Which antiemetic? J Palliat Care 1993; 9:42-50.

4. Lichter I. Results of antiemetic management in terminal illness. J Palliat Care 1993; 9:19-21.

5. Storey P. Symptom control in advanced cancer. Semin Oncol 1994; December; 21:748-753.

6. Driscoll CE. Symptom control in terminal illness. Prim Care 1987; 14:353-363.

7. Allen SG. Nausea and vomiting. In: Doyle D HG, McDonald N, ed. Oxford Textbook of Palliative Medicine. Oxford: Oxford University Press, 1993.

8. Sorey P, Knight CF. Nausea and vomiting. In: Storey P, Knight CF, eds. UNI-PAC Four: Management of Selected Nonpain Symptoms in the Terminally Ill. Gainesville: American Academy of Hospice and Palliative Medicine, 1996:39-54.

9. Ison PJ, Peroutka SJ. Neurotransmitter receptor binding studies predict antiemetic efficacy and side effects. Cancer Treat Rep 1986; 70:637-641.

10. Peroutka SJ, Snyder SH. Antiemetics: Neurotransmitter receptor binding predicts therapeutic actions. Lancet 1982; 2:658-659.

11. Schwartz RH, Beveridge RA. Marijuana as an antiemetic drug: how useful is it today? Opinions from clinical oncologists. J Addictive Disorders 1994; 13:53-65.

12. Doblin RE, Kleiman MAR. Marijuana as antiemetic medicine: A survey of oncologists' experiences and attitudes. J Clin Oncol 1991; 9:1314-1319.

13. Marsden SC. Use of ondansetron (Zofran). N Z Med J 1993; April 28:166.

14. Andrews PA, Quan V, Ogg CS. Ondansetron for symptomatic relief in terminal uraemia (letter). Nephrol Dial Transplant 1995;10:140.

15. Cole RM, Robinson F, Harvey L, Trethowan K, Murdoch V. Successful control of intractable nausea and vomiting requiring cmobined ondansetron and haloperidol in a patient with advanced cancer. J Pain Symptom Manage 1994; 9:48-50.

16. Pereira J, Bruera E. Successful management of intractable nausea with ondansetron: a case study. J Palliat Care 1996; 12:47-50.

17. Khoo D, Riley J, Waxman J. Control of emesis in bowel obstruction in terminally ill patients. Lancet 1992; 339:375-376.

18. Mercadante S, Spoldi E, Caraceni A. Octreotide in relieving gastrointestinal symptoms. Palliat Med 1993; 7:295-299.

19. Khoo D, Hall E, Motson R, Riley J, Denman K, Waxman J. Palliation of malignant intestinal obstruction using octreotide. Eur J Cancer 1994; 30A:28-30.

20. Riley J, Fallon MT. Octreotide in terminal malignant obstruction. Eur J Palliative Care 1994; 1:23-25.

21. Mangili G, Franchi M, Mariana A, Zanaboni F, Rabaiott. Octreotide in the management of bowel obstruction in terminal ovarian cancer. Gynecol Oncol 1996; 61:345-348.

22. Flynn J, Hanif N. Nabilone for the management of intractable nausea and vomiting in terminally staged AIDS. J Palliat Care 1992; 8:46-47.

23. Green ST, Nathwani D, Goldberg DJ, Kennedy DH. Nabilone as effective therapy for intractable nausea and vomiting in AIDS. Br J Clin Pharmacol 1989; 28:494-495.

24. Baines M, Oliver DJ, Carter RL. Medical management of intestinal obstruction in patients with advanced malignant disease. Lancet 1985; November 2:990-993.

25. Bruera E, Kuehn N, Miller M, et al. The Edmonton symptom assessment system (ESAS): A simple method for the assessment of palliative care patients. J Palliative Care 1991; 7:6-9.

26. Fainsinger R, Miller MJ, Bruera E, et al. Symptom control during the last week of life on a palliative care unit. J Palliat Care 1991; 7:5-11.

27. Lindley CM, Hirsch JD, O'Neill CV, Transau MC, Gilber. Quality of life consequences of chemotherapy-induced emesis. Qual Life Res 1992; 1:331-340.

28. Morrow GR. A patient report measure for the quantification of chemotherapy induced nausea and emesis: psychometric properties of the Morrow assessment of nausea and emesis (MANE). Brit J Cancer Suppl 1992;19:S72-S74.

29. Morrow GR. The assessment of nausea and vomiting. Cancer 1984; May 15; 53 Sup:2267-2278.

30. Bliss JM, Robertson B, Selby PJ. The impact of nausea and vomiting upon quality of life measures. Br J Cancer Suppl 1992; 66:314-323.

31. Melzack R, Rosberger Z, Hollingsworth M, et al. New approaches to measuring nausea. Can Med Assoc J 1985; 133:755-758.

32. Del Favero A, Roila F, Basurto C, Minotti V, Ballator. Assessment of nausea. Eur J Clin Pharmacol 1990; 38:115-120.

Nutrition and Hydration Problems in Palliative Care Patients

Kenneth C. Jackson II

SUMMARY. The provision of nutrition and hydration in terminally ill patients is controversial. Dehydration must be assessed and managed appropriately for patient comfort. Excessive hydration induces sever adverse symptoms. Oral or parenteral feeding may increase or decrease patient comfort. Contributing factors to these symptoms are discussed as are advantages and disadvantages of providing therapy. Medications associated with xerostomia are listed. Cases in which hypodermoclysis, intravenous fluid administration, and no intervention may be indicated are described. Evaluation instruments that have been used to assess the symptoms are reviewed. Some open research questions are listed. A treatment algorithm and evidence tables are presented. *[Article copies available for a fee from The Haworth Document Delivery Service: 1-800-342-9678. E-mail address: getinfo@haworthpressinc.com <Website: http://www.haworthpressinc.com>]*

KEYWORDS. Nutrition, hydration, dehydration, total parenteral, feeding, food, enteral, hypodermoclysis, intravenous, fluid, electrolytes, delirium, palliative care, terminal care, dying, supportive care, drug therapy, non-pharmacological therapy, etiologies, evidence, costs, algorithm

Kenneth C. Jackson II, PharmD, is Manager of Clinical Pharmacy Services, St. Dominic-Jackson Memorial Hospital; and Clinical Assistant Professor, University of Mississippi School of Pharmacy, Jackson, MS.

Address correspondence to: Arthur G. Lipman, PharmD, College of Pharmacy and Pain Management Center, 30 S 2000 E RM 258, University of Utah Health Sciences Center, Salt Lake City, UT 84112-5820 (E-mail: alipman@pharm.utah.edu).

[Haworth co-indexing entry note]: "Nutrition and Hydration Problems in Palliative Care Patients." Jackson, Kenneth C. II. Co-published simultaneously in *Journal of Pharmaceutical Care in Pain & Symptom Control* (Pharmaceutical Products Press, an imprint of The Haworth Press, Inc.) Vol. 8, No. 1, 2000, pp. 183-197; and: *Evidence Based Symptom Control in Palliative Care: Systematic Reviews and Validated Clinical Practice Guidelines for 15 Common Problems in Patients with Life Limiting Disease* (ed: Arthur G. Lipman, Kenneth C. Jackson II, and Linda S. Tyler) Pharmaceutical Products Press, an imprint of The Haworth Press, Inc., 2000, pp. 183-197. Single or multiple copies of this article are available for a fee from The Haworth Document Delivery Service [1-800-342-9678, 9:00 a.m. - 5:00 p.m. (EST). E-mail address: getinfo@haworthpressinc.com].

183

Algorithm for Managing Dehydration

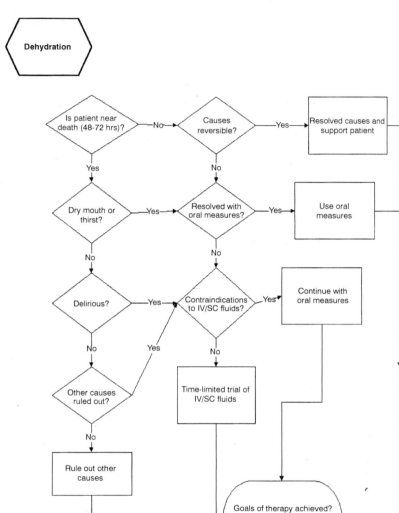

Provision of nutrition and hydration in palliative care evokes strong emotions to patients, families, and clinicians. Patients may view the use of enteral or parenteral supplementation as symbolic of their ability to survive their illness, or possibly gain extra time as they near death. Families may view provision of fluids or food as the most basic act of caring, and as such may feel it is necessary to provide these substances to their dying family member.[1] Clinicians view these modalities as tools to provide patients with comfort and improved quality of life. While use of these treatments can improve quality of life for selected patients, there are few data to support the use of enteral or parenteral therapies in most dying patients.

Dehydration and anorexia may help prepare the body for impending death.[2,3] Evidence for this is largely anecdotal in humans. Pain may result from or be exacerbated by dry mouth, thirst, or hunger. The role of hydration and nutrition is still not clear. Reports of improved cognition in patients with delirium treated for dehydration have not clarified this issue.[4]

Traditional end of life care has centered around the relief of symptoms. Treatment strategies include proving oral fluids and foods that the patient desires, as well as good oral care and hygiene. Hospice care historically has avoided the use of invasive technologies, as these therapies might be construed as over medicalizing death.[5,6] Enteral or parenteral means to supplement patients requires placement of feeding tubes, intravenous or subcutaneous catheters. Complications from these endeavors include, but are not limited to, aspiration, decreased mobility, discomfort, fluid overload, infections, and phlebitis.[7] Rectal fluid administration (proctoclysis) is another measure that has been used in hospice patients,[8] but this route is not acceptable to many patients.

PRESENTATION AND ASSESSMENT

Dehydration can be defined as the loss of normal body water.[9] Intake and output are the two main factors controlling fluid balance. The complex interaction of osmotic and hemodynamic factors control the perception of hydration status in healthy individuals. However elderly men show a tendency towards a higher threshold for the sensation of thirst in relation to dehydration.[7] Whether terminal patients have a higher threshold for thirst in relation to hydration status is unclear.

A number of factors contribute to the evaluation of dehydration in terminally ill patients. The basic evaluation should include assessments of the following:

- Input and Output (I/O's)–emphasis on inability to tolerate oral intake
- Physical examination–see below
- Symptom assessment–bed sores, constipation, delirium, decreased urinary output, thirst
- Laboratory indices–elevated BUN, creatinine, hematocrit, plasma proteins, sodium
- Review for contraindications to fluid therapy–congestive heart failure, end stage renal disease, pulmonary congestion, etc.

Physical examination of the dehydrated patient may reveal some of the following clinical features:

- Decreased skin turgor
- Dry/cracked lips and or skin
- Dysgeusia
- Muscle cramps
- Pain from dry mucosal structures or cramps
- Sunken eyes
- Xerostomia
- Xerophthalmia.

Of the physical manifestations associated with dehydration, the most distressing to patients are dry mouth, thirst, and pain. Use of oral fluids and good oral care should alleviate symptoms for most dehydrated terminally ill patients.

PROS AND CONS

Enteral or parenteral fluid or nutritional supplementation is not benign therapy. Numerous complications can result from the enteral/parenteral provision of hydration or nutrition. These complications include, but are not limited to the following:

- Agitation associated with use of medical equipment
- Ascites

- Aspiration pneumonia
- Cerebral edema
- Congestive heart failure
- Discomfort associated with tube or catheter
- Edema
- Excessive urination
- Fluid or electrolyte disorders
- Immobility associated with pump or infusion device
- Increased pulmonary secretions (increased need to cough)
- Infection at infusion site
- Leakage at infusion site
- Pericardial effusion
- Pulmonary congestion
- Trauma from placement of catheter or tube
- Vomiting–associated with increased gastrointestinal fluids.

Some patients, especially those with congestive heart failure, pulmonary disease, end stage renal or liver disease, are unable to tolerate the volume load provided by enteral or parenteral supplementation. Patients with liver damage may be unable to produce adequate levels of albumin which exacerbate the colloidal problem associated with their hydration status (i.e., ascites). Provision of TPN in these patients will not help because they are not able to make the needed albumin from the substrates provided in the TPN, TPN will worsen the fluid overload in this population.

In contrast, there are patients who will require enteral or parenteral supplementation. Terminally ill patients who require this type of supplementation fall into two categories based on life expectancy. Reasons for using these therapies differ between these two populations. Patients with a limited life expectancy who are experiencing delirium, predisposed to acute renal failure, or are refractory to other measures to relieve their dry mouth or thirst may benefit from the provision of supplemental fluids. Dehydrated terminally ill patients may experience confusion, restlessness, and neuromuscular irritability.[4,10,11] Delirium in hospice patients may be exacerbated or precipitated by accumulation of opioid metabolites due to renal insufficiency.[12] Patients with temporary intestinal obstruction may be good candidates for the provision of fluids or nutrition until the obstruction resolves.

MEDICATIONS AND XEROSTOMIA

More than 250 drugs may be responsible for causing xerostomia in patients.[13,14] Several drug classes are problematic in the palliative care population. Probably the most common problematic agents are the opioids. Additionally, certain anticonvulsants, antidepressants, anti-emetics, benzodiazepines, diuretics, and neuroleptics may be implicated in xerostomia.

Medications Known to Cause Xerostomia[1,3,22,24,25,27-31]

Class	*Selected Examples*
Opioids	morphine, methadone, oxycodone, fentanyl
Anticonvulsants	carbamazepine
Antidepressants	amitriptyline, desipramine, doxepin, fluoxetine, sertraline
Anti-emetics	metoclopramide
Anti-histamines	diphenhydramine, chlorpheniramine
Benzodiazepines	alprazolam, diazepam, triazolam
Diuretics	furosemide, hydrochlorothiazide, sprironolactone
Neuroleptics	chlorpromazine, thioridazine

EVIDENCE

A limited amount of evidence is available regarding the use of hydration or nutrition in dying patients. A compilation of the currently available literature is provided in Table 1.

Hypodermoclysis

Hypodermoclysis is the provision of fluids via the subcutaneous route. Three studies have reviewed the use of hypodermoclysis in the care of terminally ill patients. None of these studies compared patients receiving hypodermoclysis to patients receiving no parenteral fluid administration.

A retrospective analysis of 320 patients, 290 receiving hypodermoclysis and 30 receiving intravenous fluid, was performed to evaluate the daily volume of administered fluids.[11] The average daily volume for the hypodermoclysis patients was less than 50% of that administered to IV fluid patients. The authors indicated that IV fluid patients probably received excessive fluid hydration.

TABLE 1. Drug Therapy for Nutrition and Hydration Problems in Palliative Care–Evidence Table

Reference	Study Design	n	Intervention	Results	Level of Evidence	Comments
Hypodermoclysis (HDC)						
Bruera et al. (1995)[10]	Randomized double blind	25	Study population contained patients who had previously received HDC fluids as an overnight infusion. Patients received 500 mL of 2/3rd D5W and 1/3rd NS via HDC over one hour; this was repeated in 8 hours. Prior to the HDC infusion, patients received SQ hyaluronidase 150 units or 300 units. Patients were crossed over to the opposite treatment arm on day 2.	No significant differences in any variables between the two different strengths of hyaluronidase. Reasons for stopping HDC therapy were (n = 15): death (2), no longer indicated (8), SQ leakage (2), SQ bleeding (1), inadequate hydration (1), treatment refusal (1).	II	15 patients preferred 1 hour HDC, 4 preferred overnight HDC, and 6 chose to stop any further hydration.
Fainsinger et al. (1997)[15]	Prospective	100	Evaluated 100 consecutive admissions for indication of rehydration. Sixty-nine received HDC, 31 did not.	Of 69 HDC, 67 due to dehydration and 6 due to hypercalcemia (some had more than one indication). Of the 31 patients who did not get HDC, reasons were rapid deterioration and death (19), sudden death (6), and pre-existing edema and/or ascites (6).	V	Indications for using HDC: dehydration-induced delirium renal failure, increased risk of bedsores or constipation, dry mouth or thirst
Bruera et al. (1996)[11]	Retrospective	320	Reviewed 290 patients in a Palliative Care Unit (PCU) and 30 patients in a Cancer Center (CC). PCU 203/290 patients received HDC as either a continuous infusion, overnight infusion, or as three 1-hr boluses. All 30 CC patients received hydration via IV access.	PCU: HDC daily volume of 1015 +/- 135 mL/day. CC: IV daily volume of 2080 +/- 720 mL/day (p < 0.001). Authors concluded that CC patients might have received excessive amount of IV fluids.	IV	Reason for CC patients discontinuing IV fluid not available. No clear definition provided for "adequate" hydration.

TABLE 1 (continued)

Reference	Study Design	n	Intervention	Results	Level of Evidence	Comments
Intravenous fluids						
Waller et al. (1994)[16]	Prospective	68	Evaluated 68 patients (13 on IV fluids, 55 oral hydration) for state of consciousness as well as CBC and SMAC-12 results.	State of consciousness correlated with increasing sodium levels, but not necessarily route of hydration. No evidence found for unproved biochemical or clinical status with IV fluids.	III	Authors note potential selection bias with IV group.
Musgrave et al. (1995)[17]	Prospective Pilot study	30	Evaluated 19 patients with a prognosis of less than 10 days. Researchers looked at sensation of thirst, signs of fluid retention, fluid balance (I/O), and electrolyte status.	Eighteen patients (95%) experienced thirst, noted as mild (6), moderate (8), and severe (4). IV regimens ranged from 500 mL to 3000 mL per day. Thirst was not greatly influenced by IV volume administered. The 4 patients with severe thirst had no oral intake.	V	Small study without benefit of statistical analysis
Musgrave et al. (1996)[18]	Retrospective	21	Data collected on 21 patients who received IV hydration on the day of death to determine presence of rales, ascites, and swollen legs.	Rales were present 81% or patients, ascites in 62%, and leg edema in 52%. Twenty-eight percent of patients had only one sign of fluid retention, 28% had two signs, and 38% had three signs.	V	Report appears in the correspondence section of the journal.
No Intervention						
Ellershaw et al. (1995)[19]	Prospective	82	Evaluated 82 terminal patients for symptoms of dehydration. Patients were taking only sips of fluids or were no longer taking oral medications.	Only 23 patients were able to respond to questions. Of these 87% experienced dry mouth (95% CI 66-97%) and 83% expressed thirst (95% CI 61-95%). Of these patients, no significant difference was noted between patients with biochemical indices of dehydration and those with essentially normal values.	V	Authors noted that 91% of patients responding were receiving opioids.

Study	Design	N	Description		Comments
McCann et al. (1994)[22]	Prospective	32	Evaluated 32 consecutively admitted patients to a comfort care unit for presence of hunger, thirst, and dry mouth.	V	Twenty patients (63%) never experienced any hunger, while 11 patients (34%) experienced hunger only initially. In regard to thirst or dry mouth, 11 patients never experienced thirst (34%), 9 patients (28%) experienced thirst initially, and 12 patients (38%) experienced thirst until death.	All symptoms were relieved with the administration of either food and/or liquids, and provision of ice chips and mouth care. Relief lasted from one to several hours in all cases.
Burge (1993)[20]	Prospective	52	Cross sectional survey of patients to determine the severity and distribution of 7 symptoms associated with dehydration (thirst, dry mouth, bad taste, nausea, fatigue, pain, pleasure in drinking).	V	Patients distributed into two categories: high oral intake (> 750 mL/day) and low oral intake (< 750 mL/day). No association found between symptoms and oral intake or laboratory indices.	Patients did report pleasure from drinking.
Oliver (1984)[21]	Retrospective	22	Evaluated 22 hospice patients from a study on hypercalcemia in patients with advanced cancer. Patients all expired within 48 hours of venipuncture	V	Twelve patients had essentially normal electrolyte and urea panels. Five patients had elevated urea, and 5 patients had elevated calcium and urea.	Author noted the electrolyte balance was good without the use of parenteral hydration in these patients.
Case Reports					
McCann et al. (1994)[22]	Case Report	2	Report of 2 patients with thirst unrelieved by treatments for dry mouth. Treatment included artificial saliva, sips of water, use of ice chips, and treatment of oral *Candida*.	V	Patients were administered SQ normal saline and dry mouth was unproved.	No amount or duration of fluid administration was noted. Authors feel important to differentiate dry mouth from dehydration.

191

TABLE 1 (continued)

Reference	Study Design	n	Intervention	Results	Level of Evidence	Comments
Yan (1991)[23]	Case Report	3	Three patients received intermittent hypodermoclysis for GI motility disorder, severe agitation, and decreased oral intake (mild dehydration), respectively.	All three patients improved. GI problem was solved; cognitive status improved and anxiety decreased; and third patient's symptoms were controlled and discharge home was facilitated.	V	
Fainsinger and Gramlich (1997)[24]	Case Report	2	Authors report on 2 patients, out of 278 admitted over one year. Each patient was begun on TPN during admission.	Patient 1 (gastric adenocarcinoma) continued to decline despite provision of TPN. Patient continued on TPN despite medical advice to discontinue. Patient 2 (carcinoid tumor of ileum) was able to maintain weight for 7 months.	V	Authors state that TPN has a role in well-selected patient population.
Andrews et al. (1993)[25]	Case Report	3	Report on 3 patients who chose not to use/continue IV hydration or TPN.	All 3 patients able to enjoy final days without discomfort associated with fluid overload. Two of the patients had improved cognition after discontinuation of parenteral fluids.	V	None of the 3 patients experienced discomfort.
Sullivan (1993)[26]	Case Report	1	Patient had received IV fluids for 14 days. but complained of discomfort and inconvenience.	Patient died peacefully 29 days after discontinuation of IV fluids. Patient remained comfortable and lucid during entire 29 days. The patient did receive ice chips (on NG suction) on day 20 post IV discontinuation.	V	

Key to Level of Evidence classification:
Level I   Randomized trials with low false-positive (alpha) and low false-negative (beta errors); high power
Level II   Randomized trials with high false-positive (alpha) and/or high false-negative (beta errors); low power
Level III Nonrandomized concurrent cohort comparisons between contemporaneous patients who did and did not receive a given intervention
Level IV Nonrandomized historical cohort comparisons between current patients who did receive the intervention and patients (from the same institution or from the literature) who did not
Level V   Case series without control subjects

192

Hypodermoclysis appears to have been well tolerated in all three studies.[10,11,15] Hypodermoclysis was administered as a continuous infusion, an overnight infusion, or as a bolus infusion over one hour. Patient preference appears to be for the one-hour bolus infusions. Subcutaneous hyaluronidase appears to help facilitate the administration of hypodermoclysis infusions. In an evaluation of hyaluronidase 150 units versus 300 units, no significant difference was noted in the ability of patients to tolerate hypodermoclysis.[10]

Intravenous Fluid (IVF) Administration

Waller et al. evaluated 13 patients receiving IV fluids and 55 patients receiving oral hydration.[16] State of consciousness correlated with increasing serum sodium levels, but not with route of administration of fluids. No evidence was found that IV fluids improved biochemical parameters or clinical status.

Nineteen patients with a life expectancy of less than 10 days participated in a pilot study.[17] The outcome of this study was that thirst was not greatly influenced by the volume of IV fluid administered. The 4 patients who were noted to have severe thirst scores had no oral intake.

Data were published as a letter in the journal *Palliative Medicine* regarding information from 21 patients receiving IV fluids on the day of their death.[18] Patients were evaluated for signs of fluid retention, defined as rales, ascites, or leg edema. Of these patients, 28% exhibited one sign, 28% exhibited two signs, and 38% exhibited all three signs. Of the individual signs, 81% of patients presented with rales, 62% with ascites, and 52% with leg edema

No Intervention

Eighty-two patients taking small amounts of oral fluids or no longer taking oral medications were evaluated for dehydration.[19] Only 23 patients were able to respond to questions regarding their hydration status. Of those 23 patients, 87% experienced dry mouth and 83% experienced thirst. No difference was found between patients with biochemical indices of dehydration and those with essentially normal laboratory values.

The presence of dry mouth, thirst, and hunger was evaluated by

McCann and colleagues.[22] Thirty-two patients were enrolled in the study. Of these patients, 63% never experienced any hunger and 34% never experienced any thirst. Of the remaining patients, all were able to satisfy their hunger or thirst with the administration of oral food, liquids, or ice chips.

A cross sectional survey of 52 patients assessed 7 indications of dehydration, i.e., thirst, xerostomia, dysgeusia, nausea, fatigue, pain, and pleasure associated with drinking fluids.[20] Patients were stratified into two groups based on oral fluid intake of less or greater than 750 mL per day. The investigators found no association between any of the 7 indicators and the level of oral intake or laboratory indices.

Oliver reported on 22 hospice patients who were part of a larger study evaluating hypercalcemia.[21] All 22 patients died within 48 hours after venipuncture for laboratory evaluation. Interestingly, 12 patients had essentially normal electrolyte and urea panels. Five patients presented with elevated serum urea, and five patients presented with elevated serum urea and calcium. None of the 22 patients received IV fluids.

CASE REPORTS

The case reports presented in Table 1 reflect the differing approach to the management of symptoms associated with poor oral intake. However, the case reports affirm the notion that supplemental therapies must be individualized to each particular case. The use of enteral or parenteral therapies should always provide patients with comfort measures. When this cannot be accomplished, their use should be discouraged.

APPROACH TO THERAPY

The available evidence may confuse clinicians on the use of enteral or parenteral supplementation. Hopefully future research will clarify the role these therapies can play in terminally ill patients.

Selection of the appropriate approach to care should always focus on the individual patient's needs and preferences. The reader is also referred to an excellent review article by Burge.[1] Another approach to the decision analysis process is presented there.

Clinicians should be vigilant in monitoring patients for physical and psychological signs of distress. Patients with dry mouth or thirst unrelieved by oral hydration and good mouth care should be given a trial course of time-limited fluids if there are no contraindications to it. Patients unable to tolerate oral fluids, and who show signs of distress or discomfort may be candidates for parenteral fluids. Although numerous factors can cause delirium or cognitive impairment, fluid may play a vital role in re-establishing good mental function.

In contrast to fluid administration, enteral nutrition, and parenteral nutrition do not play any meaningful role in patients with impending death. These efforts almost uniformly harm patients near death. Whether or not these therapies play a role in patients with a longer life expectancy should be considered on a case by case basis.

CONCLUSION

Debate continues in regard to the use of assisted hydration and nutrition in terminally ill patients, but available evidence does give the practicing palliative care clinician some guidance. In general, decisions must be structured around both the patient's wishes and good clinical practice. Future research should more fully elucidate the role these important therapies will play in positively impacting patient care.

SOME OPEN RESEARCH QUESTIONS

1. Does subcutaneous hyaluronidase facilitate administration of fluid by hypodermoclysis?
2. Are there clinical markers that reliably indicate when hydration is no longer apt to be helpful?
3. When is total parenteral nutrition cost-effective in palliative care?

REFERENCES

1. Burge F. Dehydration and provision of fluids in palliative care. What is the evidence? Can Fam Physician. 1996;42:2383-2388.

2. Printz L. Terminal dehydration, a compassionate treatment. Arch Intern Med. 1992;152:697-700.

3. Meares C. Terminal dehydration: A review. Am J Hosp Palliat Care. 1994; 11:10-14.

4. Bruera E, Franco JJ, Maltoni M, Watanabe S, Suarez-Almazor M. Changing pattern of agitated impaired mental status in patients with advanced cancer: association with cognitive monitoring, hydration, and opiod rotation. J Pain Sympt Manage. 1995;10:287-291.

5. Chadfield-Mohr S, Byatt C. Dehydration in the terminally ill–iatrogenic insult or natural process? Postgrad Med J. 1997;73:476-480.

6. Dunphy K, Finlay I, Rathbone G, Gilbert J, Hicks F. Rehydration in palliative and terminal care: if not–why not? Palliative Medicine. 1995;9:221-228.

7. Billings J. Dehydration. In: Berger A, Portenoy R, Weissman D, eds. Principles and Practices of Supportive Oncology. Philadelphia: Lippincott-Raven; 1998: 589-601.

8. Steiner N, Bruera E. Methods of hydration in palliative care patients. J Palliat Care. 1998;14:6-13.

9. Billings J. Comfort measures for the terminally ill–Is dehydration painful? J Am Geriatr Soc. 1985;33:808-810.

10. Bruera E, de Stoutz N, Fainsinger R, Spachynski K, Suarez-Almazor M, Hanson J. Comparison of two different concentrations of hyaluronidase in patients receiving one-hour infusions of hypodermoclysis. J Pain Sympt Manage. 1995;10: 505-509.

11. Bruera E, Belzile M, Watanabe S, Fainsinger R. Volume of hydration in terminal cancer patients. Supp Care Cancer. 1996;4:147-150.

12. Fainsinger R, Bruera E. When to treat dehydration in a terminally ill patient? Supp Care Cancer. 1997;5:205-211.

13. Sreebny L, Schwartz S. A reference guide to drugs and dry mouth–2nd edition. Gerodontology. 1997;14:33-47.

14. Navazesh M. Xerostomia in the aged. Dent Clin North Am. 1989;33:75-80.

15. Fainsinger R, MacEachern T, Miller M, et al. The use of hypodermoclysis for rehydration in terminally ill cancer patients. J Pain Symptom Manage. 1994;9:298-302.

16. Waller A, Hershkovitz M, Adunsky A. The effect of intravenous fluid administration on blood and urine parameters of hydration and on state of consciousness in terminal cancer patients. Am J Hosp Palliat Care. 1994;11:22-27.

17. Musgrave C, Bartal H, Opstad J. The sensation of thirst in dying patients receiving IV hydration. J Palliat Care. 1995;11:17-21.

18. Musgrave C, Bartal N, Opstad J. Fluid retention and intravenous hydration in the dying. Palliat Med. 1996;10:53.

19. Ellershaw J, Sutcliffe J, Saunders C. Dehydration and the dying patient. J Pain Sympt Manage. 1995;10:192-197.

20. Burge F. Dehydration symptoms of palliative care cancer patients. J Pain Sympt Manage. 1993;8:454-464.

21. Oliver. Terminal Dehydration. Lancet. 1984;2:631.

22. McCann R, Hall W, Groth-Juncker A. Comfort care for terminally ill patients: The appropriate use of nutrition and hydration. JAMA. 1994;272:1263-1266.

23. Yan E. Parenteral hydration of terminally ill cancer patients. J Palliat Care. 1991;7:40-43.

24. Fainsinger R, Gramlich L. How often can we justify parenteral nutrition in terminally ill cancer patients? J Palliat Care. 1997;13:48-51.

25. Andrews M, Bell E, Smith S, Tischler J, Veglia J. Dehydration in terminally ill patients–is it appropriate palliative care? Postgrad Med. 1993;93:201-208.

26. Sullivan R. Accepting death without artificial nutrition or hydration. J Gen Int Med. 1993;8:220-224.

APPENDICES

Advances in Evidence-Based Information Resources for Clinical Practice

R. Brian Haynes

SUMMARY. Astonishing as it may be (at least to patients), it has not been possible for health care practitioners to reliably and quickly look up "current best evidence" on the management of clinical problems.

R. Brian Haynes, MD, PhD, is Professor and Chair, Department of Clinical Epidemiology and Biostatistics, Professor of Medicine, and a Member of the Health Information Research Unit at McMaster University Faculty of Health Sciences, Hamilton, Ontario, Canada, and Editor of *ACP Journal Club, Evidence-Based Medicine and Best Evidence.*

Address correspondence to: Dr. R. Brian Haynes, McMaster Health Sciences Centre, Room 2c10b, 1200 Main Street West, Hamilton, Ontario L8N 3Z5, Canada (E-mail: Bhaynes@fhs.mcmaster.ca).

Reprinted from *Journal of Pharmaceutical Care in Pain & Symptom Control* Vol. 7, No. 2, 1999, pp. 35-49. ©1999 by The Haworth Press, Inc.

[Haworth co-indexing entry note]: "Advances in Evidence-Based Information Resources for Clinical Practice." Haynes, R. Brian. Co-published in *Journal of Pharmaceutical Care in Pain & Symptom Control* (Pharmaceutical Products Press, an imprint of The Haworth Press, Inc.) Vol. 7, No. 2, 1999, pp. 35-49; and: *Evidence Based Symptom Control in Palliative Care: Systematic Reviews and Validated Clinical Practice Guidelines for 15 Common Problems in Patients with Life Limiting Disease* (ed: Arthur G. Lipman, Kenneth C. Jackson II, and Linda S. Tyler) Pharmaceutical Products Press, an imprint of The Haworth Press, Inc., 2000, pp. 199-214. Single or multiple copies of this article are available for a fee from The Haworth Document Delivery Service [1-800-342-9678, 9:00 a.m. - 5:00 p.m. (EST). E-mail address: getinfo@haworthpressinc.com].

Recently, a number of tools and services have been developed by the advocates of evidence-based health care to provide practitioners (and patients) with access to current best evidence on an expanding range of clinical topics. These include periodic print summaries of individual studies and systematic reviews of evidence, and electronic databases of reports of original studies and evidence summaries. Traditional textbooks of clinical practice are gradually being augmented or replaced by electronic versions that are more frequently updated and more often based on current best evidence. Information technology is now being harnessed to provide ubiquitous access, including at the point-of-care, to evidence-based resources. This article describes the general principles behind, and selected resources for, clinicians keeping up to date with best evidence for decision making, including a bibliography of current services. *[Article copies available for a fee from The Haworth Document Delivery Service: 1-800-342-9678. E-mail address: getinfo@haworthpressinc.com <Website: http://www.haworthpressinc.com>]*

KEYWORDS. Evidence-based health care, clinical decision-support, health technology, information technology, information retrieval, health informatics, clinical informatics, clinical epidemiology

INTRODUCTION

The health sciences journal literature contains the most current and detailed accounts of the testing of various phenomena and innovations related to health promotion and disease control and contains the best information available for the management of many health care problems. However, it is voluminous and not well organized or written for clinical application, and its use for solving clinical problems, therefore, is challenging even for the most persistent and knowledgeable clinician. In fact, most clinicians indicate that they feel overwhelmed by the literature and do not attempt to use it for solving clinical problems.[1]

Clinicians can use the clinical literature to support clinical decisions in two complementary ways: *regular surveillance* (or browsing) and *problem-oriented searches*. While the latter mode is more effective for learning, both are necessary for continuing clinical competence.

Both methods require an appreciation of the purposes of the clinical literature and a basic understanding of the strengths and weaknesses of the features of various studies for providing information that is valid and clinically applicable *for questions related to the cause, course, diagnosis, and therapy or prevention of health problems.*

CHANNELS OF COMMUNICATION
IN THE HEALTH SCIENCES LITERATURE

In general, the peer-reviewed journal literature serves science rather than clinical practice: its prime function is to provide communication from scientist to scientist[2] (Table 1). Most of the investigations reported in journals, even in "clinical" journals, are nondefinitive tests of hypotheses and innovations, only a small portion of which may eventually survive testing well enough to warrant routine clinical application.

Reports of definitive studies also appear in journals, constituting "scientist-to-clinician" communication, but these studies are in very small numbers. This situation is cause for both celebration and dismay. Celebration is in order because clinicians need to attend to only a small portion of the literature that otherwise would be far too large to manage. Dismay arises from the observation that journals scatter definitive studies among many preliminary investigations and the reader must diligently apply some basic rules of research, i.e., do a "critical appraisal," to distinguish the definitive from the preliminary studies.

Clinical review articles are published even less frequently than definitive studies. These reviews constitute clinician-to-clinician communication and the new standards that are emerging for conducting and reporting systematic reviews[3] greatly enhance the likelihood that they will provide valid conclusions based on the best available evidence.

Many journals also publish case reports and case series. While at first blush these might be considered clinician-to-clinician communications, these are perhaps best classified as clinician-to-scientist communications, as they provide ideas, based on careful observations of unplanned events, that need to be tested in planned investigations.

Finally, clinical journals also publish nonclinical scientific articles and nonscientific articles on a wide range of topics, including news,

TABLE 1. Major Channels of Communication Supported by Peer-Reviewed Clinical Journals

Channel of Communication	Types of Research Report	Relative Frequency
Scientist-to-scientist	Preliminary studies	Very high
Scientist-to-clinician	Definitive studies	Very low
Clinician-to-clinician	Systematic review articles	Very low

ethics, parables, book reviews, letters, and so on. These articles leaven the literature and add enjoyment but at an opportunity cost if they distract attention from definitive studies or mislead readers into thinking they bear definitive news for clinical practice when they don't.

CRITICAL APPRAISAL OF THE CLINICAL LITERATURE

Clinicians, themselves, can efficiently select articles from the literature that report clinically relevant and valid evidence by screening the purpose and methods of articles using principles of critical appraisal. These principles appear in brief in Table 2 and are a streamlined version of the principles that previously have been published.[4] This streamlining has been made possible by the observation that a few of the criteria can do most of the work of the full set.

Recently, a number of secondary evidence-summary publications have been developed in which studies are selected and assembled in a systematic way that includes critical appraisal of the evidence[3]. These include *ACP Journal Club, Evidence-Based Medicine, Evidence-*

TABLE 2. Guidelines for Critical Appraisal of Journal Articles

| | Topic of Study | | | | |
	Therapy	Diagnosis	Prognosis	Causation	Reviews
Criteria for Appraisal	Random allocation of patients to comparison groups	Clearly identified comparison groups, one being free of the disorder	Inception cohort, early in the course of the disorder and initially free of the outcome of interest	Clearly identified comparison group for those at risk of, or having, the outcome of interest	Comprehensive search for relevant articles
	Outcome measure of known or probable clinical importance	Objective or reproducible diagnostic standard, applied to all participants	Objective or reproducible assessment of clinically important outcomes	Masking of observers of outcome to exposure	Explicit criteria for rating relevance and merit
	Follow-up of $\geq$ 80%	Masked assessment of test and diagnostic standard	Follow-up of $\geq$ 80%	Masking of observers of exposure to outcome	Inclusion of all relevant studies

Based Cardiovascular Medicine, Evidence-Based Mental Health, and *Evidence-Based Nursing* (see Appendix for details). Clinicians can improve their efficiency in applying evidence from valid and applicable research by using these sources if the coverage of clinical content includes their field of practice.

SURVEILLANCE OF THE LITERATURE TO KEEP UP TO DATE

Regular journal reading, either first hand or through evidence-summary journals and services, is necessary to keep up to date as journals are the first peer-reviewed source of new evidence available to most clinicians. Application of critical appraisal guidelines permits definition of the journals in one's field of practice that have the highest yield of definitive articles and allows regular review of these journals at a very swift pace. For example, for all of general internal medicine and its major subspecialties, application of the guidelines identifies just 9 core journals. The yield from these journals of articles that are worthy of detailed reading by clinicians averages one article for two issues, a manageable task.

PROBLEM-ORIENTED SEARCHING OF THE CLINICAL LITERATURE

The most potent stimulus to learning in clinical practice is the unsolved problems of our patients. To use the clinical literature to help solve these problems, one must know how to search the clinical literature effectively and efficiently. The most feasible approach for most clinical disciplines *at present* is to do one's own electronic searches of the clinical literature at the time the clinical problem must be solved, employing critical appraisal guidelines to select the best articles available on the topic.[3] Because this is a demanding task, it is likely only worth doing for problems that one encounters fairly often in one's own practice.

Fortunately, there are many affordable methods of accessing the clinical literature. The most general of these is the National Library of Medicine's MEDLINE which includes citations from over 3200 journals (see Appendix). These citations are indexed with content terms and, increasingly, with methods terms (see below) that support electronic critical appraisal. Physicians can readily learn how to do searches themselves that retrieve at least as many relevant articles as the searches of trained librarians. MEDLINE is free on the internet from many sites and at least one of the free sites, PubMed, also includes pre-stored search strategies that are designed to select studies that are most likely to be relevant and valid for clinical practice (see Appendix for details). When relevant citations are retrieved, the information contained in their abstracts may be sufficient for a clinical decision to be made. When there is not enough information in the abstract, the full text of the article may be available electronically through Ovid and other online services (see Appendix).

The single best methods terms to include in MEDLINE searches to find high quality studies for clinical practice are these: "CLINICAL TRIAL (PT)" for treatments; "SENSITIVITY (TW)" for diagnostic tests; "RISK (TW)" for etiology; "EXPLODE COHORT STUDIES" for prognosis.

The Cochrane Library is now a major resource of systematic reviews and trials of health care interventions. It contains four databases, the *Cochrane Database of Systematic Reviews* (systematic reviews done by members of Cochrane Review Groups), the *Database of Abstracts of Reviews of Evidence* (other published systematic reviews), the Cochrane Controlled Trials Register (a huge database of citations of trials), and the Cochrane Review Methodology Database (citations on how to do systematic reviews).

In mid-1995, a new, more specialized type of journal-based resource became available: Best Evidence, a cumulative, electronic version of *ACP Journal Club* and *Evidence-Based Medicine,* from the American College of Physicians. This provides electronic access to all of the studies that meet reasonable criteria for scientific merit and clinical content in the major clinical fields (but not subspecialties).

In Fall 1998, Ovid released the most integrated lliterature service to date: Evidence-Based Medicine Reviews. This includes the Cochrane Database of Systematic Reviews, Best Evidence, MEDLINE, and over 200 full text journals, with cross linkages so that, for example, a search on MEDLINE that retrieves a clinical trial will provide a hypertext link to a Cochrane review or Best Evidence summary, if the trial has been reviewed by these services.

Textbooks such as *Scientific American Medicine* and *UpToDate* are beginning to support evidence-based decisions by providing extensive journal citation and frequent updating of the text. None of the existing general clinical texts, however, follows explicit standards for evidence or systematic review of evidence.

MAKING CLINICAL DECISIONS ON THE BASIS OF EVIDENCE IN JOURNAL ARTICLES

With the best available evidence at hand, the clinician is in a much better position to make an informed decision about managing the patient's problem. But it is important to note that, even at its best, evidence published in the clinical literature only answers questions such as "Does this medication, on average, do more good than harm among those who agree to take it in a clinical trial with special resources for encouraging patients and following them?" The question, "Should I prescribe this medication for this patient at this time?" is beyond the scope of clinical trials or of textbooks. Making the best decision for the patient requires sound judgement based on clinical expertise and knowledge of the patient's preferences in addition to evidence from research (see Figure 1).

We are beginning to see the emergence of evidence-based textbooks, compendia, and practice guidelines, which combine explicit and quantitative reviews of evidence with advice from those who have experience in managing the clinical problem at hand. These resources may well alleviate some of the need for practitioners to fend for themselves in accumulating, synthesizing, and interpreting evidence. Nevertheless, original evidence will almost always be published in

FIGURE 1. Basic Elements of Clinical Decision Making[5]

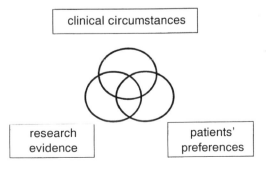

advance of synthesis, and there will always be a need for the clinician to be aware of new evidence in the management of patients. This need can only be well served if clinicians learn and apply the skills required to extract and appraise the best evidence from the literature for solving specific clinical problems.

REFERENCES

1. Williamson JW, German PS, Weiss R, Skinner EA, Bowes F III. Health science information management and continuing education of physicians. Ann Intern Med. 1989;110:151-160.

2. Haynes RB. Loose connections between peer-reviewed clinical journals and clinical practice. Ann Intern Med 1990;113:724-8.

3. Oxman AD, Guyatt GH. Guidelines for reading literature reviews. Can Med Assoc J 1988;138:697-703.

4. Sackett DL, Richardson SR, Rosenberg W, Haynes RB. Evidence-Based Medicine: how to practice and teach EBM. London: Churchill Livingstone, 1997.

5. Haynes RB, Sackett DL, Gray JRA, Cook DJ, Guyatt GH. Transferring evidence from research into practice: 1. The role of clinical care research evidence in clinical decisions. ACP J Club 1996 Nov-Dec: 125:A-14-16; Evidence-Based Medicine 1996 Nov-Dec;1:196-8. Reproduced with permission of the American College of Physicians-American Society of Internal Medicine.

APPENDIX

ANNOTATED SELECTED LIST OF RESOURCES
FOR EVIDENCE-BASED HEALTH CARE
(Information and addresses below are subject to change)

Journals

ACP Journal Club. Abstracts of articles from about 50 journals of relevance to internal medicine, the articles being selected according to critical appraisal criteria. Provided with *Annals of Internal Medicine* for American College of Physicians members, or as a separate subscription for non-members. Contact Subscriptions, ACP, tel. 800-523-1546. Available in Canada from CMA Publications, tel. 800-663-7336; and in the UK from the BMJ Publishing Group, tel. (44) 171-387-4499.

Evidence-Based Medicine. Abstracts articles from all major clinical fields (family medicine, internal medicine, obstetrics and gynecology, pediatrics, psychiatry, public health, surgery). Available by subscription from the ACP (see above), the BMJ (see above) and CMA (see above).

Evidence-Based Cardiovascular Medicine. Abstracts of relevance to cardiovascular medicine. Available from Churchill-Livingstone (Harcourt Brace; Saunders).

Evidence-Based Mental Health. Abstracts of articles of relevance to mental health care. Available from the BMJ Publishing Group (see above).

Evidence-Based Nursing. Abstracts of articles of relevance to nursing care. Available from the BMJ Publishing Group (see above), the RCN Publishing Company (tel. (44) 181-423-1066), and the Canadian Nurses Association.

Textbooks

Dixon RA, Munro JF, Silcocks PB. *The Evidence Based Medicine Workbook. Critical Appraisal for Clinical Problem Solving.* Oxford: Butterworth-Heinemann. 1997.

Eddy DM (ed). *Common Screening Tests.* Philadelphia, American College of Physicians, 1991. (Ordering: American College of Physicians, P. O. Box 7777-R-0270, Philadelphia, PA 19175, order number CDT 89.)

Friedland DJ, Go AS, Shlipak MG, Bent SW, Subak LL, Mendelson T. *Evidence-Based Medicine: A Framework for Clinical Practice.* Stamford CT: Appleton & Lange, 1998.

Haines A, Donald A (eds): *Getting Research Findings into Practice.* London: BMJ Publishing Group. 1998:78-85.

Kuhns LR, Thornbury JR, Fryback DG. *Decision Making in Imaging.* Chicago, Yearbook Medical Publishers, 1989.

Panzer RJ, Black ER, Griner PF. *Diagnostic Strategies for Common Medical Problems.* Philadelphia, American College of Physicians Press, 1991 (551 pages). (Order number DIS91 from the American College of Physicians.) (Update due in Spring 1999.)

Sackett DL, Richardson SR, Rosenberg W, Haynes RB. *Evidence-Based Medicine: how to practice and teach EBM.* London: Churchill Livingstone, 1997.

Silagy C, Haines A (eds). *Evidence Based Practice in Primary Care.* BMJ Books, BMA House, Tavistock Square, London WC1H 9JR, UK, 1998.

Sox HC Jr. (editor). *Common Diagnostic Tests. Use and Interpretation.* Second Edition. Philadelphia, American College of Physicians. 1991. (Ordering: American College of Physicians, P. O. Box 7777-R-0270, Philadelphia, PA 19175, order number CDT 89.)

Straus SE, Badenoch D, Richardson WS, Rosenberg W, Sackett DL. *Practising Evidence-Based Medicine.* Learner's Manual. 3rd Edition. Radcliffe Medical Press Ltd. Abingdon, Oxon, UK, 1998.

Computer Software

Best Evidence–cumulated contents of *ACP Journal Club* (since 1991) and *Evidence-Based Medicine* (since 1995) in an annual CD–see subscription information under *ACP Journal Club* (above). Also on the internet through Ovid (see below), with featured articles available for free at *http://acponline.org.*

The Cochrane Library–see description above. Available from Update Software. In the UK: Summertown Pavilion, Middle Way, Summertown, Oxford OX2 7LG, England (tel: +44 1865 513902 (UK), fax: +44 1865 516918, e-mail: help@update.co.uk, internet: http://update.cochrane.co.uk/). In the US: Update Software Inc., 936 La Rueda Drive Vista, CA 92084 USA, Tel: +1 760 727-6792, Fax: +1 760 734-4351, e-mail: *updateinc@home.com.* Commercial internet sites: *http://www.update-software.com/ccweb/cochrane/cdsr.htm*; *http: //www.hcn.net.au*; *http://www.medlib.com*; *http://www.ovid.com.*

SAM-CD–Scientific American *Medicine* on a compact disc and world wide web. Available from Scientific American Medicine, 415 Madison Avenue, New York, NY 10017, USA. (800-545-0554); *http://www.samed.com.*

UpToDate. Quarterly CD. Available from UpToDate Inc, 34 Washington Street #320, Wellesley MA 02181-1903, USA; tel 781-237-4788; fax781-239-0391; *http://www.uptodateinc.com.*

MEDLINE Routes

Online Systems	
Vendor	**Product**
National Library of Medicine 8600 Rockville Pike Bethesda, Maryland 20892	Internet Grateful Med: **http://igm.nlm.nih.gov/** PubMed: **http://www.ncbi.nlm.nih.gov/PubMed/clinical.html**
DIALOG Information Services, Inc. 3460 Hillview Avenue Palo Alto, California 94304	DIALOG, DIALOG Medical Connection; Knowledge Index (lowest cost per relevant citation)
Personal Bibliographic Software, Inc. P.O. Box 4250 Ann Arbor, Michigan 48106	Pro-Search–front-end software for DIALOG
Data-Star (U.S. Office) D-S Marketing, Inc. 485 Devon Park Drive, #110 Wayne, Pennsylvania 19087	Data-Star

CD ROM MEDLINE Systems	
Vendor	**Product**
OIVD (CD Plus) 333 Seventh Avenue, 6th Floor New York, New York 10001	OVID **http://www.Ovid.com/**
SilverPlatter Information, Inc. 246 Walnut St, Suite 302 Newton, MA 02160-1639	SilverPlatter–Unabridged & Clinical Subsets Also available on WWW: Physicians' Homepage, http:// **www.SilverPlatter.com/physicians**
EBSCO Electronic Information 461 Boston Road, Unit 3D Topsfield, Massachusetts 01983	EBSCO CD ROM–Unabridged & Subset
Healthcare Information Services 2335 American River Road, Suite 307 Sacramento, California 95825	BiblioMed
DIALOG Information Services, Inc. 3460 Hillview Avenue Palo Alto, California 94304	DIALOG OnDisc–Unabridged & Subset
ARIES Systems Corporation 200 Sutton Street North Andover, MA 01810	ARIES Knowledge Finder–Monthly, Quarterly & Subset (best Macintosh performance) **http://www.kfinder.com**
Evidence-filters for OVID and SilverPlatter	**http://www.ihs.ox.ac.uk/library/filters.html**

EVIDENCE-BASED MEDICINE ON THE WORLD WIDE WEB
(A sampling, with links from these to many other sites)

SHARR (links to most other EBM sites)
http://www.shef.ac.uk/uni/academic/R-Z/scharr/ir/netting.html
McMaster Health Information Research Unit http://hiru.mcmaster.ca
Oxford Centre for Evidence-Based Medicine *http://cebm.jr2.ox.ac.uk*
Cochrane Library–UK *http://www.update-software.com/clibhome/clibdemo.htm*
Cochrane Library–San Diego: *http://www.updateusa.com/clibpw/clibdemo.htm*
University of York/NHS Centre for Reviews and Dissemination (including links to
    Effective Health Care and *Effectiveness Matters*) *http://www.york.ac.uk/inst/crd/*
    dissem.htm
Evidence-Based Mental Health *http://www.psychiatry.ox.ac.uk/cebmh/*
Bandolier *http://www.jr2.ox.ac.uk/Bandolier/band50/b50-8.html*
Peds Journal Club *http://pedsccm.wustl.edu/EBJournal_club.html*
Family Practice JC (POEMS): *http://jfp.msu.edu/jclub/jc0496b.htm*
Neurosurgery *http://www.brown.edu/Departments/Neurosurgery/EJC/journ.html*
Institute for Clinical Evaluative Sciences *Informed http://www.ices.on.ca/docs/informed.*
    htm

ACP Journal Club *http://www.acponline.org/journals/acpjc/jcmenu.htm*
Evidence-Based Medicine *http://www.acponline.org/journals/ebm/ebmmenu.htm*
Best Evidence (to order in the US) *http://www.acponline.org/catalog/cbi/best_evidence. htm?ban*
Miner Library in Rochester *http://www.urmc.rochester.edu/Miner/Links/ebmlinks.html*
Biomednet *http://biomednet.com/* (free registration)
Avicenna Home Page *http://www.avicenna.com* (free MEDLINE; registration required)
Community of Science: *http://muscat.gdb.org/repos/medl* (userid and password required)
HealthGate Home Page: *http://www.healthgate.com* (registration required)
HealthWorld: *http://www.healthworld.com/Library/search/medline.htm* Guide to Best Practices: *http://www.futurehealthcare.com/pages/guidetobestpractices.htm*
Knowledge Finder *http://www.kfinder.com/* (must be registered user)
NlightN MEDLINE: *http://www.nlightn.com*

Personal Alerting Service

Institute for Scientific Information *Personal Alert.* Customized internet e-mail alerting service. ISI, 3501 Market St, Philadelphia, PA 19104, USA. Tel. 215-386-0100, 800-336-4474; Fax 215-386-2911; *HTTP://www.isinet.com.*

Journal Article on the Basics of Evidence-Based Clinical Practice

Evidence-Based Medicine. A new approach to teaching the practice of medicine. Evidence-based Medicine Working Group. JAMA 1992;268:2420-5. (EBM "call-to-arms.")

Users' Guides to the Clinical Literature Series

Guyatt GH, Rennie D. User's Guides to Reading the Medical Literature: Editorial. JAMA 1993;270(17):2096-2097.
Oxman AD, Sackett DL, Guyatt GH et al. for the Evidence-Based Medicine Working Group. User's Guides to the Medical Literature: I. How to get started. JAMA 1993;270(17):2093-2095.
Guyatt GH, Sackett DL, Cook DJ et al. for the Evidence-Based Medicine Working Group. Users' Guides to the Medical Literature: II. How to use an article about therapy or prevention A. Are the results of the study valid? JAMA 1993; 270(21):2598-2601.
Guyatt GH, Sackett DL, Cook DJ et al. for the Evidence-Based Medicine Working Group. Users' Guides to the Medical Literature: II. How to use an article about therapy or prevention B. What were the results and will they help me in caring for my patients? JAMA 1994;271(1):59-63.
Jaeschke R, Guyatt GH, Sackett DL et al. for the Evidence-Based Medicine Working Group. Users' Guides to the Medical Literature: III. How to use an article about a diagnostic test A. Are the results of the study valid? JAMA 1994;271(5):389-391.
Jaeschke R, Guyatt GH, Sackett DL et al. for the Evidence-Based Medicine Working Group. Users' Guides to the Medical Literature: III. How to use an article about a

diagnostic test B. What are the results and will they help me in caring for my patients? JAMA 1994;271(9):703-707.

Levine M, Walter S, Lee H, Haines T, Holbrook A, Moyer V for the Evidence-Based Medicine Working Group. Users' Guides to the Medical Literature: IV. How to use an article about harm. JAMA 1994;271(20):1615-1619.

Laupacis A, Wells G, Richardson S, Tugwell P for the Evidence-Based Medicine Working Group. Users' Guides to the Medical Literature: V. How to use an article about prognosis. JAMA 1994;272(3):234-237.

Oxman AD, Cook DJ, Guyatt GH for the Evidence-Based Medicine Working Group. Users' Guides to the Medical Literature: VI. How to use an overview. JAMA 1994;272(17):1367-1371.

Richardson WS, Detsky AS for the Evidence-Based Medicine Working Group. Users' Guides to the Medical Literature: VII. How to use a clinical decision analysis A. Are the results of the study valid? JAMA 1995;273(16):1292-1295.

Richardson WS, Detsky AS for the Evidence-Based Medicine Working Group. Users' Guides to the Medical Literature: VII. How to Use a clinical decision analysis B. What are the results and will they help me in caring for my patients? JAMA 1995;273(20):1610-1613.

Hayward RS, Wilson MC, Tunis SR, Bass EB, Guyatt GH for the Evidence-Based Medicine Working Group. Users' Guides to the Medical Literature: VIII. How to use clinical practice guidelines. A. Are the recommendations valid? JAMA 1995;274(7):570-574.

Wilson MC, Hayward R, Tunis SR, Bass EB, Guyatt GH for the Evidence-Based Medicine Working Group. Users' Guides to the Medical Literature: VIII. How to use clinical practice guidelines. B. What are the recommendations and will they help you in caring for your patients? JAMA 1995;274(20):1630-1632.

Guyatt GH, Sackett DL, Sinclair JC, Hayward R, Cook DJ, Cook RJ for the Evidence-Based Medicine Working Group. Users' Guides to the Medical Literature: IX. A method for grading health care recommendations. JAMA 1995;274(22):1800-1804.

Naylor CD, Guyatt GH, for the Evidence-Based Medicine Working Group. Users' Guides to the Medical Literature: X. How to use an article reporting variations in the outcomes of health services. JAMA 1996;275:554-558.

Naylor CD, Guyatt GH, for the Evidence-Based Medicine Working Group. Users' Guides to the Medical Literature: XI. How to use an article about a clinical utilization review. JAMA 1996;275(18):1435-1439.

Guyatt GH, Juniper E, Heyland DK, Jaeschke R, Cook DJ. Users' Guides to the Medical Literature: XII. How to use articles about health-related quality of life. JAMA 1997;277:1232-1237.

Drummond MF, Richardson WS, O'Brien BJ, Levine M, Heyland D. Users' Guides to the Medical Literature: XIII. How to use an article on economic analysis of clinical practice: A. Are the results of the study valid? JAMA 1997;277(19):1552-1557.

O'Brien BJ, Heyland D, Richardson WS, Drummond MF. Users' Guides to the Medical Literature: XIII. How to use an article on economic analysis of clinical practice: B. What are the results and will they help me in caring for my patients? JAMA 1997;277(22):1802-1806.

Dans A, Dans LF, Guyatt GH, Richardson S, for the EBM Working Group. Users Guides to the Medical Literature XIV. How to decide on the applicability of clinical trial results to your patient. JAMA 1998;279(7):545-549.

Systematic Review Series

Mulrow C, Cook DJ, Davidoff F. Systematic reviews: Critical links in the great chain of evidence. [Editorial] Ann Intern Med 1997;126(5):389-391.

Cook DJ, Mulrow CD, Haynes RB. Systematic reviews: Synthesis of best evidence for clinical decisions. Ann Intern Med 1997;126:376-380.

Hunt DL, McKibbon A. Locating and appraising systematic reviews. Ann Intern Med 1997;126:532-538.

Badget RG, O'Keefe MO, Henderson MC. Using systematic reviews in clinical education. Ann Intern Med 1997;126(11):886-891.

Cook DJ, Greengold NL, Ellrodt AG, Weingarten SR. The relation between systematic reviews and practice guidelines. Ann Intern Med 1997;127:210-216.

Mulrow C, Cook D. Integrating heterogeneous pieces of evidence in systematic reviews. Ann Intern Med 1997;127(11):989-995.

Lau J, Ioannidis JPA, Schmid CH. Eds: Mulrow C, Cook DJ. Quantitative synthesis in systematic reviews. Ann Intern Med 1997;127:820-826.

Meade MO, Richardson WS. Selecting and appraising studies for a systematic review. Ann Intern Med 1997;127:531-537.

Counsell C. Formulating questions and locating primary studies for inclusion in systematic reviews. Ann Intern Med 1997;127:380-387.

Bero LA, Jadad AR. How consumers and policymakers can use systematic reviews for decision making. Ann Intern Med 1997;127:37-42.

Basic Statistics for Clinicians Series

Guyatt GH, Jaeschke R, Heddle N, Cook DJ, Shannon H, Walter S. Basic Statistics for Clinicians: I. Hypothesis testing. Can Med Assoc J 1995;152:27-32.

Guyatt GH, Jaeschke R, Heddle N, Cook DJ, Shannon H, Walter S. Basic Statistics for Clinicians: II. Interpreting study results: Confidence intervals. Can Med Assoc J 1995;152:169-173.

Jaeschke R, Guyatt GH, Shannon HS, Walter SD, Cook DJ, Heddle N. Basic Statistics for Clinicians: III. Assessing the effects of treatment: Measures of association. Can Med Assoc J 1995;152:351-357.

Guyatt GH, Walter S, Shannon H, Cook DJ, Jaeschke R, Heddle N. Basic Statistics for Clinicians: IV. Regression and correlation. Can Med Assoc J 1995;152:497-504.

Health Services Research

Health Services Research Group. Standards, guidelines and clinical policies. Can Med Assoc J 1992;146:833-837.

Health Services Research Group. A guide to direct measures of patient satisfaction in clinical practice. Can Med Assoc J 1992;146:1727-17731.

Health Services Research Group. Quality of care: 1. What is quality and how can it be measured? Can Med Assoc J 1992;146:2153-2158.

Health Services Research Group. Quality of care: 2. Quality of care studies and their consequences. Can Med Assoc J 1992;147:163-167.

Health Services Research Group. Outcomes and management of health care. Can Med Assoc J. 1992;147:1775-1780.

Development of Practice Guidelines ("Guidelines for Guidelines")

Carter A. Background to the "guidelines for guidelines" series. Can Med Assoc J. 1993;148:383.

This article begins a series in the CMAJ on guidelines on the development of evidence-based practice guidelines.

The Rational Clinical Examination

This is an occasional series in the JAMA providing quantitative information on aspects of clinical examination.

Some examples:

Sackett DL. A primer on the precision and accuracy of the clinical examination. JAMA 1992;267:2645-2648.

Sackett DL, Rennie D. The science of the art of the clinical examination. JAMA 1992;267:2650-2652.

Williams JW, Simel DL. Does this patient have ascites? How to divine fluid in the abdomen. JAMA 1992;267:2645-2648.

Deyo RA, Rainville J, Kent DL. What can the history and physical examination tell us about low back pain? JAMA 1992;268:760-765.

Stephenson BJ, Rowe BH, Haynes RB, Macharia WM, Leon G. Is this patient taking the treatment as prescribed? JAMA 1993;269:2779-2781.

Williams JW, Simel DL. Does this patient have sinusitis? Diagnosing acute sinusitis by history and physical examination. JAMA 1993;270:1242-1246.

Grover SA, Barkun AN, Sackett DL. Does this patient have splenomegaly? JAMA 1993;270:2218-2221.

Sauvé JS, Laupacis A, Ostbye T, Feagan B, Sackett DL. Does this patient have a clinically important carotid bruit? JAMA 1993;270:2843-2845.

Detsky AS, Smalley PS, Chang J. Is this patient malnourished? JAMA 1994;271:54-58.

Frochling DA, Silverstein MD, Mohr DN, Beatty CW. Does this dizzy patient have a serious form of vertigo? JAMA 1994;271:385-388.

Goldstein LB, Matchar DB. Clinical assessment of stroke. JAMA 1994;271:1114-1120.

Naylor CD. Physical examination of the liver. JAMA 1994;271:1859-1865.

Kitchens JM. Does this patient have an alcohol problem? JAMA 1994;272:1782-1787.

Holleman DR, Simel DL. Does the clinical examination predict airflow limitation? JAMA 1995;273:313-319.

Siminoski K. Does this patient have a goiter? JAMA 1995;273:813-817.

Reeves RA. Does this patient have hypertension? How to measure blood pressure. JAMA 1995;273:1211-1218.

Turnbull JM. Is listening for abdominal bruits useful in the evaluation of hypertension? JAMA 1995;274:1299-1301.

Cook DJ, Simel DL. Does this patient have abnormal central venous pressure? JAMA 1996;275:630-634.

Wagner JM, McKinney WP, Carpentar JL. Does this patient have appendicitis? JAMA 1996;276:1589-1594.

Etchells E, Bell C, Robb K. Does this patient have an abnormal systolic murmur? JAMA 1997;277:564-571.

Badgett RG, Lucey CR, Mulrow CD. Can the clinical examination diagnose left-sided heart failure in adults? JAMA 1997;277:1712-1719.

Bastian LA, Piscitelli JT. Is this patient pregnant? Can you reliably rule in or rule out early pregnancy by clinical examination? JAMA 1997;278(7):586-591.

Metlay JP, Kapoor WN, Fine MJ. Does this patient have community-acquired pneumonia? Diagnosing pneumonia by history and physical examination. JAMA 1997;278(17):1440-1445.

Margolis P, Gadomski A. Does this infant have pneumonia? JAMA 1998;279(4):308-313.

Anand SS, Wells PS, Hunt D, Brill-Edwards P, Cook D, Ginsberg JS. Does this patient have deep vein thrombosis? JAMA 1998;279(14):1094-1099.

Whited JD, Grichnik JM. Does this patient have a mole or a melanoma? JAMA 1998;279(9):696-701.

The Cochrane Collaboration and Library: Accessing the Best Evidence Through Systematic Reviews

Jeanne Le Ber

SUMMARY. The Cochrane Collaboration is an international organization of individuals committed to preparing, maintaining and updating the full-text of systematic reviews, and providing access to them through the Cochrane Library. It evolved in response to Archibald Leman Cochrane's challenge to health care professionals to provide an organized summary of relevant randomized controlled trials so that treatment decisions would be made on solid evidence supported by research. There are six organizational units that comprise the Collaboration and support the work of the volunteer contributors. These units

Jeanne Le Ber, MLIS, is Assistant Librarian at the Spencer S. Eccles Health Sciences Library, University of Utah Health Sciences Center.

Address correspondence to: Jeanne Le Ber, Eccles Health Sciences Library, University of Utah Health Sciences Center, Salt Lake City, UT 84132 (E-mail: jeannele (@lib.med.utah.edu).

The author thanks Tom Oliver of the Canadian Cochrane Network and Centre for providing resources for this paper and for suggesting helpful websites, and Ted Starr of Update Software, Inc. for permission to use the screen illustrations from the Internet version of the Cochrane Library. Thanks also are extended to colleagues Wayne Peay, Joan Stoddart, and Mary Youngkin, who took the time to make suggestions about this paper.

Reprinted from *Journal of Pharmaceutical Care in Pain & Symptom Control* Vol. 7, No. 2, 1999, pp. 51-64. © 1999 by The Haworth Press, Inc.

take on various responsibilities and establish the policies, methods and guidelines for ensuring the integrity of material and data received. Available on CD-ROM and over the Internet, searching the Cochrane Library is relatively simple. *[Article copies available for a fee from The Haworth Document Delivery Service: 1-800-342-9678. E-mail address: getinfo@haworthpressinc.com <Website: http://www.haworthpressinc.com>]*

KEYWORDS. Cochrane Collaboration, Cochrane Library, history of medicine 20th century, factual databases, information storage and retrieval, systematic reviews, evidence-based medicine, randomized controlled trial

INTRODUCTION

The Cochrane Collaboration is an international, not-for-profit organization of interested individuals who participate in the production, the Cochrane Library. The Cochrane Library is an electronic full-text database accessed over the Internet by paid subscription; it is also available on diskette or CD-ROM. Included in the Cochrane Library are the full-text of systematic reviews, abstracts of reviews of effectiveness, a registry of controlled trials, and a methodology database that includes materials on the science of reviewing research.

A systematic review, as defined in the online Cochrane glossary (http://www.update-software.com/ccweb/cochrane/glossary.htm#PS), is "a review of a clearly formulated question that uses systematic and explicit methods to identify, select and critically appraise relevant research, and to collect and analyze data from the studies that are included in the review. Statistical methods (meta-analysis) may or may not be used to analyze and summarize the results of the included studies." The authors of these varied systematic reviews perform extensive searches of the scientific literature to identify and synthesize all the published and non-published studies on a specific topic. Besides being a comprehensive review of the literature, this process may reduce possible individual author bias. Criteria for producing systematic reviews are discussed later in this paper.

At a basic level, the Cochrane Library attempts to organize the medical literature so that health care providers can effectively and efficiently access the best available evidence for treatments from the research literature. As one tool for practicing evidence-based medicine, the Cochrane Library filters the current literature, thereby saving practitioners time while keeping them apprized of best current practices. David L. Sackett defined evidence-based medicine as "the conscientious, explicit and judicious use of current best evidence in making decisions about the care of individuals patients. The practice of evidence-based medicine means integrating individual clinical expertise with the best available external clinical evidence from systematic research."[1]

As an electronic database, the Cochrane Library is easily updated and amended. The individuals who contribute to the Cochrane Collaboration are committed to keeping their particular subject areas current by continuously reviewing the literature, identifying and correcting errors, and responding to valid criticism. Updated and new systematic reviews are flagged for easy identification with each quarterly revision of the library.

Academicians, health care providers, researchers and others interested in the area of pain management and symptom control, will find the Cochrane Library especially useful for reviews and references on treatment efficacy, treatment outcomes and clinical trials related to drug and pain studies. Performing a simple phrase search in the database on "drug therapy" results in nearly two-hundred systematic reviews with titles such as: *Anticonvulsants in Pain*; *Antihistamines versus Aspirin for Itch*; *Chronic Pelvic Pain in Women: All Treatments*; *Drugs versus Placebo for Dysthymia*; *Rheumatoid Arthritis: Short-term Corticosteroids*; and *Vitamin C for the Common Cold*.

The intent of this article is to provide a brief history of the Cochrane Collaboration, discuss the values and structure of the Collaboration, provide an overview of the Cochrane Library, introduce the Pain, Palliative Care and Supportive Care Group (PaPaS) and illustrate techniques for searching the Cochrane Library on the Internet.

BRIEF HISTORY OF THE COCHRANE COLLABORATION

In 1972 Archibald Leman Cochrane, a British clinician, epidemiologist and medical scientist, published *Effectiveness and Efficiency: Random Reflections on Health Services.*[2] In his book, Dr. Cochrane makes the point that physicians should be using the scientific evidence from randomized controlled trials to treat patients, and not "clinical impression, anecdotal experience, 'expert' opinion or tradition."[3] Cochrane further challenged his colleagues in 1979 when he wrote,

"It is surely a great criticism of our profession that we have not organized a critical summary, by specialty or subspecialty, adapted periodically, of all relevant randomized controlled trials." Cochrane asserted that by providing physicians access to reliable evidence, accurate and cost-effective treatment decisions for patients could be made.[4]

Iain Chalmers, a British obstetrician, responded to Cochrane's challenge by developing a comprehensive register of perinatal randomized clinical trials. Chalmers found that MEDLINE searches were inadequate for the task because so many of the clinical trials were not indexed. In addition, although articles were indexed using the medical subject headings (MeSH), they were not always indexed consistently and the earlier vocabulary lacked appropriate headings to describe controlled clinical trials. As a solution, Chalmers recruited friends and colleagues to examine the journal literature by hand-searching for published reports of perinatal trials. The results of this massive undertaking were published in 1985 in *A Classified Bibliography of Controlled Trials in Perinatal Medicine 1940-1984,* and included over 3,500 clinical trials. A regularly updated electronic version of this text was produced in 1988 as the Oxford Database of Perinatal Trials. Despite the advantages this work created for treatment decisions, Chalmers expressed concern about the comprehensiveness and accessibility of his work, as well as the fact that "published studies are a biased sample of all studies undertaken."[3]

In 1992, the British National Health Service honored Archie Cochrane by providing funds for a center, named for him, with the goal "to facilitate the preparation and maintenance of systematic reviews for all of healthcare, as had been done for the perinatal field." Iain Chalmers was appointed the first director of the Cochrane Centre. With a broad vision of the future, Chalmers encouraged the establishment of additional Cochrane Centres around the world in Denmark, Canada, Italy, the United States and Australia, and recruited individuals committed to the process of preparing and maintaining systematic reviews. By October 1993, the Cochrane Collaboration became a reality.[3]

THE VALUES AND STRUCTURE
OF THE COCHRANE COLLABORATION

In less than a decade, the Cochrane Collaboration has grown to become an international effort of tremendous scope, yet it has remained true to its initial goal of "preparing, maintaining and ensuring the accessibility of systematic reviews of the effects of health care interventions." The Collaboration espouses eight values that guide their work: collaboration, building on the enthusiasm of individuals, avoiding duplication, minimizing bias, keeping up to date, ensuring relevance, ensuring access and continually improving the quality of its work.[5]

Volunteer reviewers provide a substantial portion of the expertise, energy, time and effort to compile and maintain the Cochrane Library. Although not centrally funded, a number of agencies and organizations support the Collaboration efforts. Information about participating in the Cochrane Collaboration is available at http://www.update-software. com/ccweb/cochrane/newcomer.htm#INVOLVE. This Web page includes information about "How to Get Involved" and a "Registration of Interest" form that can be filled out online.

There are six organizational units that make up the Collaboration, providing the structure, guidelines and instructions for all the people involved:

1. *Collaborative Review Groups* (CRGs) consist of individuals who are interested in a specific health concern and are willing to contribute to the preparation of systematic reviews on their subject of interest. They work with an editorial team who gathers the material and data for submission to the Cochrane Library. As an example, members of the pharmaceutical community participate by contributing to the Cochrane Pain, Palliative and Supportive Care Group.

2. *Fields* are groupings that focus on dimensions of health, such as the setting of care, the type of consumer, the type of provider, or the type of intervention. Currently fields include such areas as the Cancer Network, Complementary Medicine, Health Care of Older People, Health Promotion, Primary Health Care, Rehabilitation and Related Therapies, and Vaccines.

3. *Cochrane Centres* do the administrative work that keeps the system working. The Centres keep directories of interested reviewers, bring people with similar subject interests together, coordinate review group searching of the literature, develop Collaboration guidelines and software, and organize outreach services.

4. *Methods Working Groups* establish the guidelines that reviewers follow as they organize, prepare, analyze and present their systematic reviews. *The Reviewer's Handbook* is available online at http://www.medlib.com/cochranehandbook/ or it can be downloaded in one of a number of formats (Macintosh or PC) at http://www.update-software.com/ccweb/cochrane/hbook.htm.
5. *Consumer Network* encourages the consumer (patient, family and others) to become involved in the process of the Collaboration by providing input and feedback.
6. *Cochrane Collaboration Steering Group* (CCSG) consists of members selected from review groups, the consumers network, Cochrane Centres and Fields. The CCSG governs and sets policies for the Collaboration.[6]

Collaboration is the operative word, and each of these units performs a necessary function for the success of the whole.

OVERVIEW OF THE COCHRANE LIBRARY

Updated quarterly, the Cochrane Library is available to subscribers on diskette (there are currently 21 diskettes but this product is being phased out), CD-ROM, and over the Internet. In the United States, Update Software, Inc. (http://www.UpdateUSA.com) works closely with the Collaboration and produces the software and Internet interface for searching the Cochrane Library.

Different from a bibliographic database such as MEDLINE, the Cochrane Library contains quality-assessed information. Reviewers include meta-analyses of similar interventions when appropriate and possible, and provide access to the resulting charts and graphs with the reviews. The Cochrane Library contains four separate databases:

1. *The Cochrane Database of Systematic Reviews* contains original systematic reviews done by members of the Collaborative Review Groups.
2. *Database of Abstracts of Reviews and Effectiveness* (DARE) contains structured abstracts of systematic reviews that have been critically appraised by reviewers.
3. *The Cochrane Controlled Trials Register* is a bibliographic database of controlled trials.

4. *The Cochrane Review Methodology Database* is a bibliography of articles on the science of research synthesis.

In addition, the Cochrane Library contains information about the Cochrane Collaboration and the process of developing the database, and software updates. There are links to *The Reviewer's Handbook,* an online instruction manual on the science of reviewing research, as well as links to the Collaborative Review Groups, Methods Working Groups, Networks, and sources of support.

Producing a systematic review is a very structured process with very specific criteria. Each review contains a brief statement of its objectives, the search strategy used to review the literature, the selection criteria for including studies, data collection and analysis, main results, and conclusions. The main body of the review includes all the details related to the brief statements, as well as tables, charts and references. Users of the Cochrane Library need to develop a critical eye to determine the validity of the systematic reviews, and to determine whether they will be helpful with their practice. In a recent article, Hunt and McKibbon[7] list eight questions people should ask when assessing the quality of a systematic review; these are listed in Table 1.

PAIN, PALLIATIVE CARE AND SUPPORTIVE CARE GROUP

Registered in January 1998, the Pain, Palliative Care and Supportive Care Group (PaPaS) currently has over 200 volunteer members. As stated on their website (http://www.jr2.ox.ac.uk/Cochrane/), the

TABLE 1. Questions to ask when assessing the quality of a systematic review.

1. Did the review article address a focused question?
2. Is it likely that important, relevant studies were missed?
3. Were the inclusion criteria used to select articles appropriate?
4. Was the validity of the included studies assessed?
5. Were the assessments of studies reproducible?
6. Were the results similar from study to study?
7. What are the overall results and how precise are they?
8. Will the results help in caring for patients?[7]

PaPaS concentrates their efforts in the area of interventions concerned with the following three points:

- Prevention and treatment of acute and chronic pain
- Relief of symptoms resulting from the disease process or interventions used in the management of disease and symptom control
- Supporting patients and their caregivers through the disease process

This group has prepared and continues to maintain a systematic review on *Anticonvulsant drugs for the management of acute and chronic pain,* as well as protocols for *Acupuncture for chronic headache,* and *Corticosteroids for the resolution of bowel obstruction.* Additional topics covered by the collaborative review group include ethical issues for treatment and palliative care, psychological preparation for painful medical procedures, symptoms associated with pain and palliative care, control of post-operative pain, relaxation in chronic pain, chronic pain, treatments for migraine, and cognitive behavioral therapy.

Interested individuals can contact Frances Fairman, the PaPaS Review Group Coordinator, at:

Pain, Palliative & Supportive Care CRG
Pain Relief Unit
The Churchill Hospital
Oxford OX3 7LJ UK
Phone: 44 1865 225762;
Fax: 44 1865 225400
E-mail: frances.fairman@pru.ox.ac.uk

SEARCHING THE COCHRANE LIBRARY ON THE INTERNET

Searching the Cochrane Library on the Internet is relatively easy. Each search screen has a toolbar at the top with eight icons that represent various functions such as exit, databases, records, feedback (not yet implemented at the time this was written), export, help, and previous 25 records and next 25 records. This toolbar allows the database user to move between screens and within documents. Search terms are entered in the search text box just below the toolbar.

Searches can be initiated from any screen that contains the text box. The help icon links to the online instruction manual that describes techniques for searching and browsing the Cochrane Library, using MeSH (medical subject headings), and tips on refining search strategies. An options link provides the opportunity to limit retrieval with date and field restrictions.

SEARCHING WITH TEXT WORD

Enter a term in the search text box and then click on the search button. The system defaults to searching for the term in the title, abstract, author name, citation, and keyword fields. In addition, text words can be truncated with the asterisk; this retrieves all possible suffixes of a root word (e.g., typing *pain**, retrieves records with the word(s) pain, pains, pained, painful, painless, etc.). Word case, punctuation, numbers and words less than 3 characters are ignored by the system. Boolean operators AND, OR, NOT, and proximity operators NEXT or NEAR, are not indexed and are used only for combining or restricting searches. The options link allows text words to be limited to specific fields (title, author, abstract, or keyword), as well as date. When performing the text word query, all databases in the Cochrane Library are searched, and the results displayed in a database table. Databases and their sub-sections are listed on the left, with the number of records retrieved by the search, called hits, on the right. Click on the left link to view retrieved records.

The Figure 1 example (using a screen from the 1998 Issue 3 of the Cochrane Library) illustrates a text word phrase search for information on *pain management*. The phrase is put in quotes so the system searches for that specific phrase and not articles dealing with pain AND management, which would give slightly different results.

The results of the above search are displayed in Figure 2. Note that

FIGURE 1. Initial Phrase Search for Pain Management

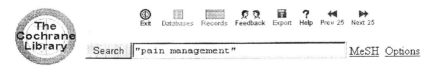

FIGURE 2

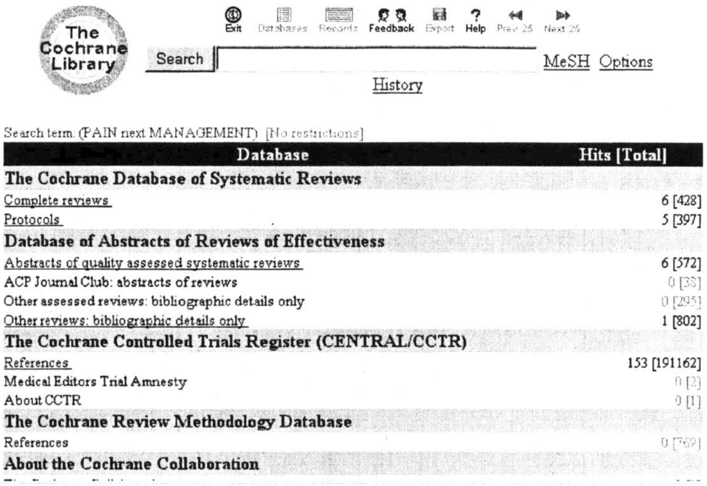

the numbers of complete reviews, protocols, abstracts of quality assessed systematic reviews, bibliographic details and references are displayed in the right column. (The number in brackets equates with the total number of hits in the entire database.) View records by clicking on the appropriate link on the left side of the screen.

As an example of Cochrane Library content, the six full-text titles listed under complete reviews in the Cochrane Database of Systematic Reviews include: (1) *Anticonvulsants in pain*; (2) *EMLA to reduce circumcision pain*; (3) *Patient education for neck pain*; (4) *Sucrose for pain in neonates*; (5) *Support during childbirth*; (6) *TENS/ALTENS effectiveness in chronic low back pain*. Depending on the information need, one or more of these reviews may prove helpful.

The five records listed under the protocols link deal with (1) *Behavioral treatment for chronic LBP*; (2) *Chronic pain in venous leg ulcers*; (3) *Exercise therapy for low back pain*; (4) *Multidisciplinary teams in chronic LBP*; and (5) *Spinal manipulation for low back pain*. Similarly, by exploring the links under Abstracts of Reviews of Effectiveness and the Cochrane Controlled Trials Register additional lists of resources are available.

SEARCHING WITH MEDICAL
SUBJECT HEADINGS (MESH)

There are three steps involved when searching the Cochrane Library with medical subject heading: (1) choosing an initial MeSH heading from the permuted index; (2) selecting the MeSH heading to search on; and (3) searching on the chosen term.

Enter a term in the text box then click on the MeSH link directly to the right. From the displayed list, click on the appropriate MeSH term. Move both up and down through the tree structure to select either a more general or more specific terms. To move up or down a level in a MeSH tree, click to highlight a term above or below the current term. The tree display will be re-drawn with the newly selected term in red.

With the selected term shown in red, click again to highlight that term. At this point, there is the option to do a single term search (to search for only the term shown in red) or to explode the term (search on the term in red and all of the terms listed underneath that term). Search results are specific to the medical subject heading selected.

An example of the initial MeSH search screen is reproduced in Figure 3. In this case the thesaurus term being searched is *pain*. By clicking on a more specific MeSH term, for instance back-pain or pain-measurement, a second screen, Figure 4, displays the tree structure and provides the option to perform a singe term search or use the explode capability.

LIST OF THE MESH VOCABULARY
THAT RELATES TO PAIN

Additional Search Features

Search terms can be combined using the Boolean operators AND, OR, NOT, and adjacency operators NEAR, NEXT. The Boolean operator AND is the default and individual words entered without operators will be AND'ed together. Listed below are examples of Boolean and adjacency operator searches:

- Entering *pain AND management* retrieves records that contain both these words.

- Entering *pain AND (management OR treatment)* retrieves records that contain the word pain, associated with either the word management or the word treatment.
- The operator NEXT links the words or phrases on either side of the word. Entering *pain NEXT management* is the same as "*pain management,*" except the word order is not specified.
- The operator NEAR performs the same function as NEXT, but instead of retrieving words that are exactly next to each other, it searches on words within six words of each other. Entering *pain NEAR management* retrieves sources that include statements such as management decisions related to control of pain, or management or treatment options for severe pain.

FIGURE 3. Entering a Term in the MeSH Thesaurus

Exit	Databases	Records	Feedback	Export	Help	Prev 25	Next 25

Thesaurus   pain

FIGURE 4

PAIN
    ABDOMINAL-PAIN
    ACUTE-PAIN-SERVICE see PAIN-CLINICS
    ANALOGUE-PAIN-SCALE see PAIN-MEASUREMENT
    BACK-PAIN
    CHEST-PAIN
    FACIAL-PAIN
    LOW-BACK-PAIN
    MCGILL-PAIN-QUESTIONNAIRE see PAIN-MEASUREMENT
    MULTIDISCIPLINARY-PAIN-CENTERS see PAIN-CLINICS
    MYOFASCIAL-PAIN-SYNDROMES
    NECK-PAIN
    PAIN
    PAIN-CLINICS
    PAIN-INSENSITIVITY-CONGENITAL
    PAIN-MEASUREMENT
    PAIN-THRESHOLD
    PAIN-INTRACTABLE
    PAIN-POSTOPERATIVE
    PAIN-ASSESSMENT see PAIN-MEASUREMENT

Search History

The Cochrane Library system software keeps track of every search entered in the text box. Click on history and then click on a search statement to initiate retrieval and view results. When viewing the history, search statements can be recombined by entering the pound sign and the search statement number in the search text box. All numbered searches can be erased from history by clicking on the clear button. Figure 5 illustrates the history options.

CONCLUSION

Archie Cochrane was the impetus that spurred the creation of the Cochrane Collaboration and the ensuing production of the Cochrane Library. Providing access to systematic reviews of controlled trials and other evidence, the Cochrane Library is an excellent resource for healthcare providers searching for the best evidence for health care interventions. Contributors to the Collaboration are committed to reviewing and updating their work. Users' of the Cochrane Library are encouraged to send their comments and criticisms to collaborative review group authors in order to maintain the integrity of the information provided in the database. Individuals interested in working with the Collaboration can fill out a registration of interest form online at http://www.update-software.com/ccweb/cochrane/newcomer.htm.

FIGURE 5. History Options

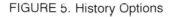

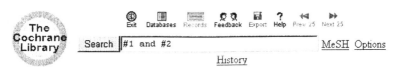

The Cochrane Library just recently became available over the Internet and provides relatively easy methods for searching.

Subscribing to the Cochrane Library

Internet access to the Cochrane Library is available from Update Software, Inc. for a subscription fee. This company works closely with the Cochrane Collaboration and other groups interested in gathering and reviewing research evidence to produce electronic publications, specialized research registers, and tools for synthesizing the results of clinical research. For more information on Update Software, Inc., or the Cochrane Library, contact: Update Software, Inc. 936 La Rueda Drive/ Vista, California 92084; Phone: 1-760-727-6792; Fax: 1-760-734-4351; E-mail: updateinc@home.com or info@updateusa.com; Website: http://www.UpdateUSA.com

REFERENCES

1. Sackett, DL, Richardson, WS, Rosenberg, W, Haynes, RB. Evidence-based Medicine: How to practice and teach EBM. New York: Churchill Livingstone, 1997.

2. Cochrane AL. Effectiveness and efficiency: Random reflections on Health Services. London: Nuffield Provincial Hospitals Trust; 1972.

3. Dickersin K, Manheimer E. The Cochrane Collaboration: evaluation of health care and services using systematic reviews of the results of randomized controlled trials. Clin Obstet Gynecol 1998; 41(2):315-31.

4. Chalmers I. The Cochrane collaboration: preparing, maintaining, and disseminating systematic reviews of the effects of health care. Ann NY Acad Sci 1993; 703:156-63; discussion 163-5.

5. Collaboration Collaboration. Cochrane Brochure. Available online at http://hiru.mcmaster.ca/cachrane/cochrane/cc-broch.htm; July 2, 1998.

6. Jadad AR, Haynes RB. The Cochrane Collaboration–advances and challenges in improving evidence-based decision making. Med Decis Making 1998; 18(1):2-9.

7. Hunt DL, McKibbon KA. Locating and appraising systematic reviews. Ann Intern Med 1997; 126(7):532-8.

Index

A Classified Bibliography of Controlled Trials in Perinatal Medicine 1940-1984, 218

Abdominal muscle tone, decreased, constipation due to, 50

Absorbable collagen sheet hemostat (INSTAT), for cancer-related bleeding, 43t,44

Absorbable collagen sponge (Helistat), for cancer-related bleeding, 43t

Absorbable gelatin sponge (Gelfoam), for cancer-related bleeding, 40t,41t,43t,44

Abuse, substance, depression and, 76

ACE inhibitors
  dysgeusia due to, 153
  xerostomia due to, 152

ACE inhibitors/lithium, delirium due to, 62

Acetaminophen, for dyspnea, 119

ACP Journal Club, 204

Acquired immunodeficiency syndrome (AIDS)
  cachexia in, 11
  diarrhea in, 96,99
  enteric protozoal infections in, diarrhea due to, 97
  viral infections in, diarrhea due to, 97

Activity, decreased, constipation due to, 50

Acyclovir
  delirium due to, 62
  depression due to, 76

Agency for Health Care Policy and Research (AHCPR), of the Public Health Service, U.S. Department of Health and Human Services, 6

Aggressive oral hygiene therapy, in oral mucositis prevention, 146

Agra, Y., 56

Ahmedzai, S., 123

AIDS. *See* Acquired immunodeficiency syndrome

Akathasia, drug-induced, 26

Albuterol (Proventil, Ventolin), for dyspnea, 118t

Alkylating agents, for mucositis, 155

Alopecia, megestrol acetate and, 20

Alprazolam (Xanax)
  for anxiety, 28-29,30,31t,32t
  for nausea and vomiting, 176

Altretamine, delirium due to, 62

Alzheimer's disease, depression and, 76

Amantadine, delirium due to, 62

American College of Critical Care Medicine, in anxiety management, 29

Aminocaproic acid, for cancer-related bleeding, 40t,42t,44

Aminophylline, for dyspnea, 118t

Amitriptyline
  for depression, 74t,80,82t,83t,84t
  for mucositis, 133

Amoxapine, for depression, 81,84t

Amoxicillin, for mucositis, 155

Amphetamine-like drugs, depression due to, 76

Anabolic steroids, depression due to, 76

Anemia, fatigue due to, 132

Anesthesia/anesthetics, local
  for dyspnea, 117t
  inhaled, for dyspnea, 122-123
  for oral mucositis, 147

Anger, depression and, 76
Anhedonia, depression and, 76
Anileridine, for dyspnea, 113t
Anorexia
    AIDS-associated, megestrol acetate
        for, 19
    constipation due to, 49
    evaluation of, 20-21
    fatigue due to, 133
    in palliative care patients, 11-22
        management of, 13-20,14t-18t
            algorithm for, 12
            drugs in, 13-20,14t-18t. See
                also Drug(s), for
                anorexia and
                cachexia
            supportive therapy in, 13
            underlying cause in, 13
        research questions related to, 21
Anorexia/cachexia syndrome,
        cancer-related,
        metoclopramide for, 20
Anthracene(s), for mucositis, 155
Antianxiety agents, for nausea and
        vomiting, 176
Antibiotic(s)
    antitumor, for mucositis, 155
    dysgeusia due to, 153
    fluoroquinolone, depression due to,
        76
Anticholinergic agents
    delirium due to, 62
    for dyspnea, 117t,121-122
Anticonvulsant(s)
    depression due to, 76
    xerostomia due to, 152,188
Antidepressant(s)
    for anxiety, 29
    for depression, 79-81,82t-86t,87
    dysgeusia due to, 153
    tricyclic, for depression,
        78-87,82t-86t
    xerostomia due to, 152,188
Antiemetic(s), xerostomia due to,
        152,188
Antihistamine(s)

delirium due to, 62
    for nausea and vomiting, 174
    xerostomia due to, 152,188
Antihyperlipidemic(s), dysgeusia due
        to, 153
Antihypertensive(s), dysgeusia due to,
        153
Anti-inflammatory drugs
    nonsteroidal (NSAIDs)
        depression due to, 76
        dysgeusia due to, 153
        xerostomia due to, 152
    nonsteroidal/lithium, delirium due
        to, 62
Antimetabolite(s), for mucositis, 155
Antineoplastic agents, delirium due to,
        62
Antiparkinsonian drugs, dysgeusia
        due to, 153
Antipsychotic(s), atypical, for anxiety,
        30
Antitumor antibiotics, for mucositis,
        155
Antiviral agents, dysgeusia due to,
        153
Anxiety
    in cancer patients
        categories of, 26
        sources of, 25,26
    diarrhea due to, 97
    with dyspnea, in palliative care
        patients, 111
    fatigue due to, 132, 133
    in palliative care patients, 23-35
        causes of, 25-26
        drugs and, 26
        management of
            algorithm for, 24
            drugs in, 27-30,31t-33t. See
                also specific drugs
            muscle relaxation in, 28
            non-pharmacological, 27
        presentation of, 26
        research questions related to, 30
        symptoms of, 26
            drugs associated with, 27

pathological, defined, 25
Apathy, depression and, 76
Appetite, loss of, with dyspnea, in
    palliative care patients, 111
Asacol. *See* Mesalamine
L-Asparaginase, delirium due to, 62
Asparaginase, depression due to, 76
Aspirin
    for diarrhea, 100t,105t
    for nausea and vomiting, 172t
Ativan. *See* Lorazepam
Atropine
    delirium due to, 62
    for dyspnea, 117t,122
Atrovent. *See* Ipratropium bromide
Avitene. *See* Microfibrillar collagen
    hemostat
Azathioprine, for mucositis, 155

Baclofen, depression due to, 76
Bacterial infection, diarrhea due to, 97
Barbiturate(s), depression due to, 76
Beck Depression Inventory, 77
Beckwith, M.C., 47
Benzodiazepine(s)
    for anxiety, 29
    depression due to, 76
    dysgeusia due to, 153
    for dyspnea, 117t,121,124
    short-acting, for anxiety, 28
    xerostomia due to, 152,188
Best Evidence, 204
Beta sympathetic agents, for dyspnea,
    123
Beta-adrenergic blockers, depression
    due to, 76
Beta-blockers, xerostomia due to, 152
Beta-lactam antibiotics, delirium due
    to, 62
Bisacodyl, for constipation, 54t,55
    opioid-induced, 53
Bismuth subsalicylate (PeptoBismol),
    for diarrhea, 105t
Bleeding problems

cancer-related, management of
    drugs in, 39-45,40t-43t. *See
    also specific drug*
in palliative care patients, 37-46
    causes of, 39
    management of
        algorithm for, 38
        supportive care in, 39
    research questions related to, 45
Bleomycin, delirium due to, 62
H$_2$-Blockers, dysgeusia due to, 153
Bosmin, gauze packing with, for
    cancer-related bleeding, 41t
Bowel
    compression in, constipation due
        to, 50
    tumor in, constipation due to, 50
Brain malignancy, delirium due to, 61
Breitbart, W., 29
Bristol-Myers Anorexia/Cachexia
    Recovery Instrument
    (BACRI), 21
Bromocriptine
    delirium due to, 62
    depression due to, 76
Bronchodilator(s)
    dysgeusia due to, 153
    for dyspnea, 118t
Bruera, E., 116,120,139
Bupivicaine, for dyspnea, 122-123
Bupropion (Welbutrin)
    delirium due to, 62
    for depression, 80-81,82t,85t
Burge, F., 194
Buspar. *See* Buspirone
Buspirone (Buspar)
    for anxiety, 29,33t
    for dyspnea, 124
Butyrophenone(s), for nausea and
    vomiting, 169

Cachexia
    in AIDS patients, 11
    evaluation of, 20-21
    fatigue due to, 133
    in palliative care patients, 11-22

management of, 13-20,14t-18t
  algorithm for, 12
  research questions related to, 21
Calcium channel blockers
  dysgeusia due to, 153
  xerostomia due to, 152
Calcium-channel blockers, depression
    due to, 76
Calvary Hospital, New York City, 3
Campbell, M., 121
Cancer
  anxiety in patients with, sources of,
    25,26
  CNS, depression and, 76
  constipation in patients with,
    management of, 56
  depression and, 76
  in palliative care patients
    diarrhea and, 96,99
    dyspnea and, 111
    fatigue and, 131
  pancreatic, depression and, 76
Cancer-related anorexia-cachexia
    syndrome, metoclopramide
    for, 20
Cannabinoid(s), for nausea and
    vomiting, 175,179
Capsaicin, for oral mucositis, 147
Carafate. *See* Sucralfate
Carbamazepine
  delirium due to, 62
  for mucositis, 155
Carcinoid syndrome, diarrhea due to,
    97
Cardiac glycosides, xerostomia due to,
    152
Caries, in palliative care patients, 151
Carmustine, delirium due to, 62
Casanthranol, docusate with, for
    constipation, 54t
Celexa. *See* Citalopram
Cella, D.F., 21
Cellulose
  oxidized, for cancer-related
    bleeding, 40t,43t,44

oxidized regenerated, for
    cancer-related bleeding,
    43t,44
Central nervous system (CNS),
    metastases to, delirium due
    to, 61
Cerebrovascular disease, depression
    and, 76
Chalmers, I., 218
Chambers, M.S., 143
Chemotherapy
  for dyspnea, 115
  mucositis due to, 148,154-156
  nausea and vomiting due to,
    177-179
Chloral hydrate, delirium due to, 62
Chlorpromazine (Thorarine)
  for anxiety, 29
  anxiety due to, 26
  for delirium, 64,66t-68t,69
  for dyspnea, 113t,117t,122
  for nausea and vomiting, 166t,169
Chlorpromazine (Thorazine), for
    anxiety, 32t
Chochinov, H.M., 77
Cholestyramine, for diarrhea, 100t
Cholestyramine powder (Questran,
    Prevalite), for diarrhea, 105t
Christopher's Hospice, London,
    England, 4
Cimetidine, delirium due to, 62
Ciprofloxacin, for mucositis, 155
Cisapride, for nausea and vomiting,
    175
Cis-platinum, delirium due to, 62
Citalopram (Celexa, Remeron), for
    depression, 79-80,83t,84t
Citrucel. *See* Methylcellulose
Clinical literature
  clinical decisions based on,
    205-206,205t
  critical appraisal of, 202-203,202t
  problem-oriented searching of,
    203-205
  surveillance of, 203

Clinical practice, evidence-based information resources for, advances in, 199-206

Clomipramine, for depression, 80

Clonidine, depression due to, 76

CNS. *See* Central nervous system

Coagulation protein defects, bleeding problems associated with, 39

Cochrane, A.L., 217,227

Cochrane Collaboration and Library accessing best evidence through systematic reviews in, 215-228

    introduction to, 216-217

    history of, 217-218

    on internet, searching of, 222-227, 223f,224f,226f,227f

    list of vocabulary that relates to pain, 225-227,227f

    with MESH, 225, 226f

    with text word, 223-224,223f, 224f

    overview of, 220-221

    structure of, 218-220

    values of, 218-220

Cochrane Collaboration Steering Group (CCSG), 220

Cochrane Controlled Trials Register, 204

Cochrane Database of Systematic Reviews, 204

Cochrane Review Methodology Database, 204

Codeine, for dyspnea, 119

Codeine sulfate, for diarrhea, 105t

Cognitive exercises, for depression, 77

Cohen, M., 120

Colace. *See* Docusate

Colic, abdominal, laxatives and, 53

Colitis, ulcerative, diarrhea due to, 97

Collagen, INSTAT, for cancer-related bleeding, 40t

Collagen absorbable hemostat (INSTAT), for cancer-related bleeding, 44

Communication, in health sciences literature, channels of, 201-202,201t

Compliance, poor, depression and, 76

Conill, C., 131

Connecticut hospice, 4

Constipation

    cancer-induced, management of, 56

    defined, 49

    evaluation of, 49

    opioid-induced, management of, 51t-52t,53,54t

    in palliative care patients, 47-57

    causes of, 47,49-50

    evaluation of, 49

    management of

    algorithm for, 48

    drugs in, 50-57,51t-52t,54t. *See also specific drug*

    goal of, 56

    supportive care in, 50

    prevalence of, 56

    prevention of, 53

    research questions related to, 57

    vincristine-induced, 56

Cooperation, lack of, depression and, 76

Corticosteroid(s)

    for anorexia and cachexia, 18t,19

    delirium due to, 62

    depression due to, 76

    for dyspnea, 115,117t,122

    for fatigue, 134,135t-136t,138t

    for nausea and vomiting, 175-176,179

Coyle, N., 132

Crowther, A.G.O., 55

Cryotherapy

    for mucositis, 158t

    in oral mucositis prevention, 146

Cyclizine, for nausea and vomiting, 167t,174

Cyclobenzaprine, for mucositis, 155

Cycloserine, depression due to, 76

Cylert. *See* Pemoline

Cyproheptadine (Periactin)

for anorexia and cachexia,
15t,18t,20
for diarrhea, 105t
Cyproterone, depression due to, 76
Cystosine arabinoside, delirium due
to, 62

Dapsone, depression due to, 76
*Database of Abstracts of Reviews and
Effectiveness (DARE)*, 220
*Database of Abstracts of Reviews of
Evidence*, 204
"Dear Heath Professional letter," 78
Decadron. *See* Dexamethasone
Defecation, frequency of, 49
Dehydration, fatigue due to, 132,133
Delirium
defined, 61
described, 61
in palliative care patients, 59-70
causes of, 61-62
challenges from, 61
management of
algorithm for, 60
attention to underlying
source in, 62
chlorpromazine in,
64,66t-68t
confusion related to, 61
drugs in, 63-65,66t-68t,69
haloperidol in, 64,66t-68t,69
lorazepam in, 66t-68t,69
midazolam in, 64,66t,68t,69
non-pharmacologic, 63
propofol in, 65,68t,69
presentation of, 59
research questions related to, 69
terminology related to, 61
vs. dementia, 61
Dementia
HIV, depression and, 76
vs. delirium, 61
Depression
constipation due to, 50

with dyspnea, in palliative care
patients, 111
fatigue due to, 132,133
in palliative care patients, 71-89
acceptance as normal, problems
related to, 73
anger in, 76
apathy in, 76
cancer and, 76
CNS, 76
diagnosis of, unreliability of
available tools in, 77
drugs and, 76
identification of, 73,76-77
incidence of, 73
lack of cooperation in, 76
management of
algorithm for, 72
antidepressants in, 79-81,
82t-86t,87
drugs in, 74t-75t,76,77-87,
82t-86t
non-pharmacologic, 77
psychostimulants in,
78-79,87
psychotherapy in, 77
TCAs in, 80-81,82t-86t,87
mood changes in, 76
pancreatic cancer and, 76
poor compliance in, 76
psychological stress with, 73
research questions related to, 87
social withdrawal in, 76
substance abuse and, 76
symptoms of, 76
Deseryl. *See* Trazodone
Desipramine (Norpramine), for
depression, 80,82t,83t,84t
Dexamethasone (Decadron)
for anorexia and cachexia, 14t
delirium due to, 62
for dyspnea, 117t
for fatigue, 135t
for nausea and vomiting,
166t,170t,173t,175
Dexedrine. *See* Dextroamphetamine

Dextroamphetamine (Dexedrine)
for depression, 78-79,82t
for fatigue, 139
Dextroamphetamine (Dexedrine), for
depression, 86t
Diarrhea
acute, in palliative care patients,
management of, algorithm
for, 92
in AIDS patients, 96,99
chronic, in palliative care patients,
management of, algorithm
for, 93
defined, 96
in hospice patients, 96,99
infection-induced, in palliative care
patients, management of,
algorithm for, 94
laxative-induced, in palliative care
patients, management of,
algorithm for, 95
megestrol acetate and, 20
in palliative care patients, 91-108
cancer and, 96,99
causes of
evaluation of, 96
treatment of, 97
management of
drugs in, 100t-106t
supportive therapy in, 98-99
prevalence of, 96,99
research questions related to, 99
Diazepam (Valium)
for anxiety, 32t
for depression, 75t
for dyspnea, 117t,121
Diclofenac, for mucositis, 155
Dietary fiber, inadequate intake of,
constipation due to, 49
Diflunisal, for mucositis, 155
Digitalis glycosides, depression due
to, 76
Digoxin, delirium due to, 62
Dimenhydrinate, for nausea and
vomiting, 166t,167t

Diphenhydramine, for nausea and
vomiting, 174
Diphenoxylate/atropine (Lomotil), for
diarrhea, 105t
Diprivan. *See* Propofol
Disopyramide, depression due to, 76
Disseminated intravascular
coagulation (DIC), bleeding
problems associated with, 39
Disulfiram/metronidazole, delirium
due to, 62
Disulfiram, depression due to, 76
Diuretic(s)
dysgeusia due to, 153
for dyspnea, 118t,123
thiazide, depression due to, 76
xerostomia due to, 152,188
Diuretic(s)/lithium, delirium due to,
62
Docusate (Colace, Doxidan
Peri-Coalce, Therevac-SB), for
constipation, 54t
Peri-Colace, Therevac-SB)
with casanthranol, for
constipation, 54t
in constipation prevention,
53
in glycerin base minienema,
for constipation, 54t
Docusate sodium/glycerin
mini-enemas, for
constipation, 55
Dolasetron, for nausea and vomiting,
174
Dopamine antagonists, for nausea and
vomiting, 169,174
Doxepin, for depression,
80,82t,83t,84t
Doxepram, for dyspnea, 123
Doxidan. *See* Docusate
Dronabinol (Marinol)
adverse effects of, 20
for anorexia and cachexia, 15t,18t
Droperidol, for nausea and vomiting,
174
Drug(s). *See also specific drug*

for anorexia and cachexia,
13-20,14t-18t
corticosteroids, 18t
cyproheptadine, 15t,18t
dexamethasone, 14t
dronabinol, 15t,18t
hydrazine sulfate, 15t
interferon α_{2b}, 17t
megestrol acetate, 16t,17t,18t
methylprednisolone, 14t
metoclopramide, 18t
pentoxifylline, 15t
prednisolone, 14t
research questions related to, 21
for anxiety, 27-30. *See also specific
drug*
anxiety due to, 26
for cancer-related bleeding,
39-45,40t-43t. *See also
specific drug*
for constipation, 50-57,51t-52t,54t.
See also specific drug
delirium due to, 61,62
for dementia, 63-65,66t-68t,69
for depression,
74t-75t,76,77-87,82t-86t
depression due to, 76
for diarrhea, 100t-106t
for dyspnea,
112t-113t,116-124,117t-118t
fatigue due to, 133
for mucositis, 158t
for nausea and vomiting, 166t-167t
for nutrition and hydration
problems, 188
oral complications due to, 151
withdrawal from, anxiety due to,
26
for xerostomia, 188
Drug withdrawal, depression and, 76
Drug-drug interactions, delirium due
to, 62
Dry mouth. *See* Xerostomia
Ducusate, with senna, for
constipation, 54t
Dysgeusia

defined, 168
in palliative care patients,
151,153-154
Dysphagia, in palliative care patients,
151
Dysphoric mood, depression and, 76
Dyspnea
megestrol acetate and, 20
in palliative care patients,
109-127
anxiety and, 111
assessment of, measurement
tools in, 124-125
cancer and, 111
causes of, evaluation of,
111,114-115
depression and, 111
fatigue and, 111
loss of appetite and, 111
management of
algorithm for, 110
anticholinergic agents in,
121-122
benzodiazepines in, 121,124
beta sympathetic agonists in,
123
chemotherapy in, 115
chlorpromazine in, 122
corticosteroids in, 115,122
diuretics in, 123
drugs in, 112t-113t,116-124,
117t-118t
local anesthetics in, 122-123
opioids in, 119-121
oxygen in, 116-119,117t-118t
phosphodiesterase inhibitors
in, 123
promethazine in, 122
radiation therapy in, 115
supportive therapy in,
115-116
underlying cause in,
111,114-115
onset of, 115
pain and, 111
pathophysiology of, 111

research questions related to, 125

sleep disorders and, 111

symptoms of, 111

Edema, peripheral, megestrol acetate and, 20

Educational interventions, for depression, 77

Effectiveness and Efficiency: Random Reflections on Health Services, 217,218

Effexor. *See* Venlafaxine

Electroconvulsive therapy (ECT), for depression, 77

Electrolyte abnormalities, delirium due to, 61

Emotional support, for depression, 77

Enalapril, for mucositis, 155

Encephalopathy(ies), metabolic, delirium due to, 61

Enema(s)
  for constipation, 51t,55
  sodium phosphate/sodium biphosphate enema, for constipation, 54t,55

Enteral feeding, diarrhea due to, 97

Enteric protozoal infections, in AIDS patients, diarrhea due to, 97

Environmental factors, delirium due to, 61

Erythema, mucositis and, 148

Erythromycin, for mucositis, 155

Escalante, C., 111

Estrogen(s), depression due to, 76

Evacuation, manual, for constipation, 51t,55

Evidence
  as basis for palliative care. *See* Palliative care, evidence-based
  and palliative care, 5-6

Evidence-based health care, annotated selected list of resources for, 207-214

Evidence-based information resources, for clinical practice, advances in, 199-206

Evidence-Based Medicine, 204

Evidence-based medicine, defined, 3

Exercise(s)
  cognitive, for depression, 77
  fatigue due to, 133

Fairman, F., 222

Farncombe, M., 120

Fatigue
  defined, 131
  with dyspnea, in palliative care patients, 111
  in palliative care patients, 129-141
    anemia and, 132
    anorexia and, 133
    anxiety and, 132,133
    cachexia and, 133
    cancer and, 131
    causes of, 132-133
    evaluation of, 133
  components of, 131-132
  dehydration and, 132,133
  depression and, 132,133
  diagnosis of, 132
  drugs and, 133
  exercise and, 133
  fever and, 133
  hypercalcemia and, 133
  hypoxia and, 133
  infections and, 132,133
  insomnia and, 133
  management of, 132-133
    algorithm for, 130
    drugs in, 134-139,135t-138t
    supportive therapy in, 133-134
    underlying cause in, 133
  mechanisms of, 131-132
  metabolic diseases and, 133

pain and, 132-133
prevalence of, 131
research questions related to, 139
Fecal impaction, diarrhea due to, 97
Fentanyl, for dyspnea, 120
Fever, fatigue due to, 133
Fibrinolysis, primary, bleeding
        problems associated with, 39
Fibrinolytic inhibitors, for
        cancer-related bleeding, 44
5000 lux wide-spectrum white light,
        for depression, 74t
Fleets enema. *See* Sodium
        phosphate/sodium
        biphosphate enema
Fludarabine, delirium due to, 62
Fluid intake, inadequate, constipation
        due to, 49
Fluoroquinolone antibiotics,
        depression due to, 76
5-Fluorouracil (5-FU), delirium due
        to, 62
Fluoxetine
        for depression, 79,80,83t,84t
        for mucositis, 155
Fluphenazine, for nausea and
        vomiting, 169
Flurazepam, for depression, 75t
Furosemide (Lasix), for dyspnea, 118t,
        123

Ganciclovir, delirium due to, 62
Gastrointestinal system,
        radiation-induced damage to,
        diarrhea due to, 97
Gelfoam, for cancer-related bleeding,
        40t,41t,43t,44
Gianturco wire coils, for
        cancer-related bleeding, 40t,
        42t
Glucocorticoid(s), for dyspnea, 122
Glycerin rectal suppositories, for
        constipation, 54t
Glycophyrrole, for dyspnea, 122
Glycoside(s)

cardiac, xerostomia due to, 152
digitalis, depression due to, 76
Granisetron, for nausea and vomiting,
        174,179
Greenhalgh, T., xiv
Guilt, feelings of, depression and, 76

Halitosis, in palliative care patients,
        151
Haloperidol
        for anxiety, 29
        anxiety due to, 26
        for delirium, 64,66t-68t,69
        for nausea and vomiting, 166t,167t,
        170t,173t,174
Haloperidol/carbamazepine, delirium
        due to, 62
Haloperidol/lithium, delirium due to,
        62
Haloperidol/methyldopa, delirium due
        to, 62
Harris, A.C., 55
Haynes, R.B., 199
Health care, evidence-based,
        annotated selected list of
        resources for, 207-214
Health sciences literature,
        communication in, channels
        of, 201-202,201t
Helistat. *See* Absorbable collagen
        sponge
Helplessness, depression and, 76
Hematological abnormalities, delirium
        due to, 61
Hemorrhage, oral, in palliative care
        patients, 151
Hemostatic agents, topical, for
        cancer-related bleeding,
        44-45
Higginson, I., xv,111
Histamine $_1$/muscarinic receptor
        blockers, for nausea and
        vomiting, 174
HIV. *See* Human immunodeficiency
        virus

HMG-COA reductase inhibitors, depression due to, 76
Holland, J.C., 28
Hopelessness, feelings of, depression and, 76
Hormonal agents, dysgeusia due to, 153
Hospice patients, diarrhea in, 96,99
Hospice programs
  Connecticut, 4
  in United States, number of, 4
Hospital Anxiety and Depression Scale, 77
Human immunodeficiency virus (HIV) dementia, depression and, 76
Hunt, D.L., 221
Hydration
  hypodermoclysis in, 188,193
  impaired, in palliative care patients, 151
  problems related to, in palliative care patients, 183-197
    assessment of, 185-186
    case reports, 194
    management of
      algorithm for, 184
      approach to, 194-195
      complications of, 186-187
      drugs in, 188
      intravenous fluids in, 193
      literature related to, 188-194, 189t-192t
    no intervention in, 193-194
    presentation of, 185-186
    research questions related to, 195
Hydrazine sulfate, for anorexia and cachexia, 15t,20
Hydrocortisone, for diarrhea, 105t
Hydromorphone, for dyspnea, 113t,119-120
Hydroxyurea, delirium due to, 62
Hydroxyzine (Vistaril), for anxiety, 29,32t

Hyoscine, for nausea and vomiting, 166t,174
Hyoscyamine, for dyspnea, 117t,122
Hypercalcemia
  constipation due to, 50
  fatigue due to, 133
Hyperglycemia, megestrol acetate and, 20
Hypodermoclysis, 188,193
Hypogeusia, defined, 168
Hypokalemia, constipation due to, 50
Hypothyroidism, constipation due to, 50
Hypoxia
  delirium due to, 61
  fatigue due to, 133

Ibuprofen, for mucositis, 155
Ifosfamide, delirium due to, 62
Imipramine, for depression, 80
Imodium. *See* Loperamide
Impotence, megestrol acetate and, 20
Indomethacin, delirium due to, 62
Infection(s)
  bacterial, diarrhea due to, 97
  delirium due to, 61
  depression and, 76
  diarrhea due to, in palliative care patients, management of, algorithm for, 94
  fatigue due to, 132,133
  in palliative care patients, 151
  viral, in AIDS patients, diarrhea due to, 97
Information resources, evidence-based, for clinical practice, advances in, 199-206
Insomnia, fatigue due to, 133
INSTAT collagen, for cancer-related bleeding, 40t,43t,44
Interferon(s)
  delirium due to, 62
  INF-α, depression due to, 76

INF-α_{2b}, for anorexia and
  cachexia, 17t
Interleukin-2, delirium due to, 62
Internet, Cochrane Library on,
  searching of, 222-227,
  223f,224f,226f,227f
Intestinal obstruction, constipation
  due to, 50
Intravenous fluids, 193
Ipratropium bromide (Atrovent), for
  dyspnea, 118t
Irish Sisters of Charity, Dubin,
  Ireland, 3
Irritable bowel syndrome, diarrhea
  due to, 97
Isobutyl-2-cyanoacrylate, for
  cancer-related bleeding,
  40t,44,45
Ison, P.J., 165
Isotretinoin, depression due to, 76

Jackson, J.M., 55
Jackson, K.C., II, 23,59,71,143,183
Jamjian, M.C., 37

Kaolin, pectin, and attapululgite
  suspension (Kaopectate), for
  diarrhea, 105t
Kaolin/pectin suspension, for diarrhea,
  105t
Kaopectate, for diarrhea, 105t
Ketoprofen, for mucositis, 155
Ketorolac, for mucositis, 155

Lactulose
  for constipation, 51t,52t,54t,55-56
  in constipation prevention, 53
Lasix. *See* Furosemide
Laxative(s)
  bulk-forming, in constipation
    prevention, 53
  for constipation, 51t-52t,53-57,54t

diarrhea due to, in palliative care
  patients, management of,
  algorithm for, 95
  overuse of, diarrhea due to, 97
  stimulant, for opioid-induced
    constipation, 53
Le Ber, J., 215
Lederle, F.A., 56
Levodopa, depression due to, 76
Levoprome. *See* Methotrimeprazine
Lichter, I., 165
Lidocaine (Xylocaine)
  delirium due to, 62
  for dyspnea, 117t,122-123
  viscous, for mucositis, 158t
Light, white, for depression, 74t
Lipase (Pancrease), for diarrhea, 105t
Lipman, A.G., xi-xii,1,11,23,59,129
Lloyd, S., 21
Lomotil. *See* Diphenoxylate/atropine
Loperamide (Imodium), for diarrhea,
  106t
Loprinzi, C.L., 19,134
Lorazepam (Ativan)
  for anxiety, 30,32t
  for delirium, 66t-68t,69
  for dyspnea, 121
  for nausea and vomiting, 166t,176
Lovastatin, for mucositis, 155
Lynn, J., 111
Lyophilized dura mater, for
  cancer-related bleeding, 40t

Macroscopic brain pathology,
  depression and, 76
Maguire, P., 28
Malabsorption, diarrhea due to, 97
Malignancy, brain, delirium due to, 61
Management of Cancer Pain, 6
Manual evacuation, for constipation,
  51t,55
MAO inhibitors/SSRIs, delirium due
  to, 62
MAOIs, for depression, 81-82,86t
MAOIs/SSRIs, delirium due to, 62

Maprotiline, for depression, 81,85t
Marinol. *See* Dronabinol
Martin, A.C., 71
Mast cell stabilizers, dysgeusia due to, 153
McCann, R., 194
McKibbon, K.A., 221
Meclizine, for nausea and vomiting, 166t
Medication(s). *See* Drug(s)
MEDLINE, National Library of Medicine's, 203-204
Mefloquine, depression due to, 76
Megace. *See* Megestrol acetate
Megestrol acetate (Megace)
    adverse effects of, 20
    in AIDS-associated anorexia, 19
    for anorexia and cachexia, 16t,17t,18t
    for fatigue, 134,135t 136t,138t
    initial dose of, 19
    in patients with demonstrated weight loss, 19
Mellaril. *See* Thioridazine
Menstrual irregularities, megestrol acetate and, 20
Mesalamine (Pentasa, Asaco), for diarrhea, 106t
MESH, searching Cochrane Collaboration and Library on internet with, 225, 226f
Metabolic disorders, fatigue due to, 133
Metabolic encephalopathy, delirium due to, 61
Metamucil. *See* Psyllium mucilloid
Methotrexate, delirium due to, 62
Methotrimeprazine (Levoprome)
    for anxiety, 29,33t
    anxiety due to, 26
    for nausea and vomiting, 167t
Methylcellulose (Citrucel)
    in constipation prevention, 53
    for diarrhea, 106t
Methyldopa
    delirium due to, 62

depression due to, 76
Methyldopa/lithium, delirium due to, 62
Methylphenidate (Ritalin), 75t
    for depression, 78-79,82t,86t,87
    for fatigue, 137t,138t,139
Methylphenydate (Ritalin), for dyspnea, 123
Methylprednisolone
    for anorexia and cachexia, 14t
    for fatigue, 135t,136t
Metoclopramide (Reglan)
    for anorexia and cachexia, 18t
        cancer-related, 20
    anxiety due to, 26
    depression due to, 76
    for nausea and vomiting, 166t, 167t,170t,174,175
Metrizamide, depression due to, 76
Metronidazole, depression due to, 76
Mexilitine, delirium due to, 62
Microfibrillar collagen hemostat (MCH), for cancer-related bleeding, 43t
Midazolam (Versed)
    for anxiety, 33t
    for delirium, 64,66t,68t,69
    for dyspnea, 121
Milk of magnesia, for constipation, 54t
Minagawa, H., 73
Mitazapine, for depression, 81,82t, 85t
Modified Medical Research Council Dyspnea Scale and Oxygen Cost Diagram, 124
Monoamine oxidase inhibitors (MAOIs), for depression, 81-82,86t
Monoamine oxidase inhibitors (MAOIs)/SSRIs, delirium due to, 62
Mood(s), dysphoric, depression and, 76
Mood changes, depression and, 76
Mor, V.M., 165

Morphine
   for dyspnea, 112t-113t,117t,
      119-121
   for mucositis, 158t
Motor restlessness, drug-induced, 26
Mucositis
   chemotherapy-induced, in
      palliative care patients,
      154-156
   defined, 147
   differential diagnosis of, 147
   oral
      described, 146
      in palliative care patients,
         143-161
         chemotherapy and, 148
         drugs and, 151
         erythema and, 148
         management of, 146-157
            algorithm for, 145
            categories of, 146
            drugs in, 158t
            general considerations in,
               156-157
         non-cancer patients, 150
         prevention of, 146
            algorithm for, 144
         radiation therapy and,
            148-149
         research questions related to,
            157
Muscle relaxants, dysgeusia due to,
      153
Muscle relaxation, for anxiety, 28
Muscle tone, abdominal, decreased,
      constipation due to, 50
Muscle trismus, in palliative care
      patients, 151
Myodil, for cancer-related bleeding,
      40t

Nabilone
   for dyspnea, 123
   for nausea and vomiting, 167t
Nabumetone, for mucositis, 155

Naloxone
   for cancer-induced constipation, 56
   for constipation, 51t,52t
   for dyspnea, 121
Naproxen, for mucositis, 155
Nardil. *See* Phenelzine
National Library of Medicine's
      MEDLINE, 203-204
Nausea, megestrol acetate and, 20
Nausea and vomiting
   chemotherapy-induced, literature
      related to, 177-179
   evaluation of, 176-179
   in palliative care patients, 163-181
      causes of, evaluation of, 165
      literature related to, 177-179
      management of
         algorithm for, 164
         antianxiety agents in, 176
         cannabinoids in, 175,179
         corticosteroids in,
            175-176,179
         defining of, 168
         dopamine antagonists in,
            169,174
         drugs in, 166t-167t
         general, 168
         histamine$_1$/muscarinic
            receptor blockers
            in, 174
         octreotide in, 176
         prokinetic agents in, 175
         serotonin receptor
            antagonists in,
            174-175
         underlying causes in, 168
         useful strategies in, 169-176,
            170t-173t
      research questions related to,
         179
Nefazodone (Serzome), for
      depression, 81,83t,85t
Neuroleptic(s), xerostomia due to,
      152,188
Newton's third law of motion, 4
Nicotine polacrilex, for mucositis, 155

Nicotine replacement, dysgeusia due to, 153
Norfloxacin, for mucositis, 155
Norpramine. *See* Desipramine
Nortriptyline
  for depression, 74t,75t,80,82t, 83t,84t
  for mucositis, 155
NSAIDs
  depression due to, 76
  dysgeusia due to, 153
  xerostomia due to, 152
NSAIDs/lithium, delirium due to, 62
Nu-Knit. *See* Oxidized regenerated cellulose
Nutritional status, impaired
  delirium due to, 61
  in palliative care patients, 151,183-197
    assessment of, 185-186
    case reports, 194
    management of
      algorithm for, 184
      approach to, 194-195
      complications of, 186-187
      drugs in, 188
      intravenous fluids in, 193
      literature related to, 188-194, 189t-192t
    no intervention in, 193-194
    presentation of, 185-186
    research questions related to, 195

Octreotide (Sandostatin)
  for diarrhea, 100t-101t,106t
  for nausea and vomiting, 166t,176
Ofloxacin, for mucositis, 155
Olanzapine, for anxiety, 30
Oliver, 194
Ondansetron, for nausea and vomiting, 166t,174,179
Oozing, in palliative care patients, 37-46. *See also* Bleeding problems, in palliative care patients

Opioid(s)
  constipation due to, management of, 51t-52t,53-57,54t
  delirium due to, 62
  depression due to, 76
  dysgeusia due to, 153
  for dyspnea, 112t-113t,117t, 119-121
  for mucositis, 158t
    oral, 147
  for nausea and vomiting, 172t
  xerostomia due to, 152,188
Opium tincture, for diarrhea, 106t
Oral cavity, evaluation of, in palliative care patients, 147
Oral hemorrhage, in palliative care patients, 151
Oral hygiene therapy, in oral mucositis prevention, 146
Oral mucosa
  problems associated with, in palliative care patients, 143-161. *See also* Mucositis, oral, in palliative care patients
  structural damage to, in palliative care patients, 151
Osteoradionecrosis, in palliative care patients, 151
Oxidized cellulose (Oxycel), for cancer-related bleeding, 40t,43t,44
Oxidized regenerated cellulose (Nu-Knit,Surgicel), for cancer-related bleeding, 43t,44
Oxycodone, for dyspnea, 119
Oxygel. *See* Oxidized cellulose
Oxygen, for dyspnea, 112t,116-119, 117t-118t

Pain
  depression and, 76
  with dyspnea, in palliative care patients, 111

fatigue due to, 132,133
Palliative Care and Supportive
    Care Group (PaPaS),
    221-222,221t
in palliative care patients, 151
Palliative care
    barriers to, 4-5
    defined, 3
    evidence and, 5-6
    evidence-based, 1-9
        algorithms in, 8
        historical background of, xiii
        limitations of, xiv
        questions related to, xiv-xv
        modern, evolution of, 3-4
        quality of life measurements in, xiv
        symptom prevalence in, 7
Palliative care patients. *See also under*
    each symptom or disorder
    anorexia in, 11-22
    anxiety in, 23-35
    bleeding in, 37-46
    cachexia in, 11-22
    constipation in, 47-57
    delirium in, 59-70
    depression in, 71-89
    diarrhea in, 91-108
    dysgeusia in, 153-154
    dyspnea in, 109-127
    fatigue in, 129-141
    hydration problems related to,
        183-197
    nausea and vomiting in, 163-181
    nutrition problems related to,
        183-197
    oral cavity examination in, 147
    oral complications in, 150-157
    oral mucositis in, 143-161
    xerostomia in, 151-153
Palliative Care Unit at Royal Victoria
    Hospital, Montreal, Canada, 4
Pamate. *See* Tranylcypromine
Pancrease. *See* Lipase
Pancreatic cancer, depression and, 76
Paraneoplastic syndromes, delirium
    due to, 61

Paroxetine (Paxil), for depression,
    79,83t,84t
Paxil. *See* Paroxetine
Pemoline (Cylert), for depression,
    75t,78-79,82t,86t
Penicillamine, for mucositis, 155
Penicillin
    delirium due to, 62
    for mucositis, 155
Pentasa. *See* Mesalamine
Pentoxifylline, for anorexia and
    cachexia, 15t,20
PeptoBismol. *See* Bismuth
    subsalicylate
Pergolide, depression due to, 76
Periactin. *See* Cyproheptadine
Peri-Colace. *See* Docusate
Peripheral edema, megestrol acetate
    and, 20
Peroutka, S.J., 165
Phenelzine (Nardil), for depression, 86t
Phenergan. *See* Promethazine
Phenothiazine(s)
    for dyspnea, 117t
    for nausea and vomiting, 169
Phenylpropanolamine, depression due
    to, 76
Phenytoin/lithium, delirium due to, 62
Phosphodiesterase inhibitors, for
    dyspnea, 123
Piroxicam, for mucositis, 155
Plant alkaloids/synthetic derivatives,
    for mucositis, 155
Platelet dysfunction, bleeding
    problems associated with, 39
Posture, poor, constipation due to, 50
Prednisolone
    for anorexia and cachexia, 14t
    for fatigue, 136t
Prednisone
    delirium due to, 62
    for dyspnea, 117t,122
    for nausea and vomiting, 175
Prevalite. *See* Cholestyramine powder
Primary fibrinolysis, bleeding
    problems associated with, 39

Problem-solving therapy, for depression, 77
Procarbazine
    delirium due to, 62
    depression due to, 76
Prochlorperazine
    anxiety due to, 26
    for nausea and vomiting, 167t,169,174
Progesterone agents, for dyspnea, 123
Progestin(s), depression due to, 76
Prokinetic agents, for nausea and vomiting, 175
Promethazine (Phenergan)
    for dyspnea, 117t,122
    for nausea and vomiting, 166t,170t,172t,174
Propofol (Diprivan), 65,68t,69
    for anxiety, 33t
Protein defects, coagulation, bleeding problems associated with, 39
Proton pump inhibitors, dysgeusia due to, 153
Protozoal infecitons, enteric, in AIDS patients, diarrhea due to, 97
Proventil. *See* Albuterol
Psychostimulant(s), for depression, 78-79,87
Psychotherapy, for depression, 77
Psyllium, in constipation prevention, 53
Psyllium mucilloid (Metamucil), for diarrhea, 106t
Purine antagonists, for mucositis, 155

Quality of life, in palliative care patients, measurement of, xiv
Questran. *See* Cholestyramine powder
Quinidone, delirium due to, 62
Quinolone(s), delirium due to, 62

Radiation therapy
    for dyspnea, 115
    mucositis due to, 148-149

Radiation-induced gastrointestinal damage, diarrhea due to, 97
Ranitidine, delirium due to, 62
Rash(es), megestrol acetate and, 20
Razavi, D., 26
H_2-Receptor blockers, depression due to, 76
Rectal suppositories, glycerin, for constipation, 54t
Reglan. *See* Metoclopramide
Relaxation, muscle, for anxiety, 28
Remeron. *See* Citalopram
Respiridone, for anxiety, 30
Restlessness
    motor, drug-induced, 26
    terminal, in palliative care patients, 61
Reuben, D.B., 165
Richardson, A., 131
Ritalin. *See* Methylphenidate
Roenen, J., 21
Roth, A.J., 29
Royal Victorian Hospital, Montreal, Canada, 4

Saliva, in maintaining integrity of teeth and oral mucosa, 149
Sandostatin. *See* Octreotide
Saquinavir, delirium due to, 62
Saunders, C., xiii,4
Schnell, H.W., 19
Scientific American Medicine, 204-205
Scopolamine
    for dyspnea, 122
    for nausea and vomiting, 167t,174
Seizure(s), delirium due to, 61
Selective serotonin reuptake inhibitors (SSRIs), for depression, 78-87,82t-86t
Selegine, delirium due to, 62
Self-esteem, loss of, depression and, 76
Senna
    for constipation, 51t,52t,54t,55,56,57
    docusate with, for constipation, 54t
    for opioid-induced constipation, 53

Senokot. *See* Senna
Senokot-S. *See* Docusate, with senna
Sepsis, delirium due to, 61
Serotonin receptor antagonists, for
     nausea and vomiting,
     174-175
Sertraline (Zoloft), for depression,
     79,83t,84t
Serzome. *See* Nefazodone
Short-term, defined, 29
Sialorrhea, in palliative care patients,
     151
Social support, for depression, 77
Social withdrawal, depression and, 76
Society of Critical Care Medicine, in
     anxiety management, 29
Sodium phosphate/sodium biphosphate
     enema (Fleets enema), for
     constipation, 54t,55
Sokot. *See* Senna
Sorbitol
     for constipation, 52t,54t,56
     in constipation prevention, 53
SSRIs. *See* Selective serotonin
     reuptake inhibitors
Steatorrhea, diarrhea due to, 97
Steroid(s)
     anabolic, depression due to, 76
     dysgeusia due to, 153
Stiefel, F., 26
Stomatitis
     defined, 147
     in palliative care patients, 146
     treatment of, 147
Stone, P., 131
Stool softening agents, in constipation
     prevention, 53
Storey, P., 121
Substance abuse, depression and, 76
Sucralfate (Carafate)
     for mucositis, 158t
     for oral mucositis, 147
Suicidal ideation, depression and, 76
Sulfasalazine, for mucositis, 155
Sulfonamide(s), depression due to, 76
Suppositories

for constipation, 51t
     rectal, glycerin, for constipation,
        54t
Surgicel. *See* Oxidized regenerated
     cellulose
Sykes, N.P., 56
Symptom(s), in dying patients,
     prevalence of, 7
Symptom control, evidence-based
     approach to, historical
     background of, xiii

Tamoxifen, depression due to, 76
Taxane(s), for mucositis, 155
TCAs. *See* Tricyclic antidepressants
Terminal restlesness, in palliative care
     patients, 61
Tetracycline, for mucositis, 155
*The Cochrane Controlled Trials
     Register*, 220
*The Cochrane Database of Systematic
     Reviews*, 220
*The Cochrane Review Methodology
     Database*, 221
The Reviewer's Handbook, 220,221
Theophylline, for dyspnea, 118t
Therevac-SB. *See* Docusate
Thiazide diuretics, depression due to, 76
Thioridazine (Mellaril)
     for anxiety, 29,33t
     for delirium, 68t
     for depression, 74t
Thorazine. *See* Chlorpromazine
Thrombin (Thrombostat,
     Thrombogen), for
     cancer-related bleeding, 43t
Thrombin sponges, for cancer-related
     bleeding, 44
Thrombocytopenia, bleeding problems
     associated with, 39
Thrombogen. *See* Thrombin
Thrombosis, venous, megestrol
     acetate and, 20
Thrombostat. *See* Thrombin
Tocainide, delirium due to, 62

Toilet access, inconvenient, constipation due to, 50
Topiramate, delirium due to, 62
Tranexamic acid, for cancer-related bleeding, 40t,42t,44
Tranylcypromine (Pamate), for depression, 86t
Trazodone (Deseryl), for depression, 81,83t,85t
Triazolam, for mucositis, 155
Tricyclic antidepressants (TCAs), for depression, 78-87,82t-86t
Trimethoprim/sulfamethoxazole (TMP-SMZ), for mucositis, 155
Trimetrexate, for mucositis, 155
Trimipramine, for depression, 80,84t
Trismus, muscle, in palliative care patients, 151
Tumor(s)
    in bowel wall, constipation due to, 50
    vasoactive intestinal peptide, diarrhea due to, 97
Tyler, L.S., 11,109,129,163

Ulcer(s), in palliative care patients, 151
UpToDate, 204-205

Valium. *See* Diazepam
Valproic acid, delirium due to, 62
Varricchio, C.G., 131
Vascular defects, bleeding problems associated with, 39
Vasoactive intestinal peptide tumor (VIPoma), diarrhea due to, 97
Venlafaxine (Effexor), for depression, 81,83t,85t
Venous thrombosis, megestrol acetate and, 20
Ventafridda, V., 122
Ventolin. *See* Albuterol
Versed. *See* Midazolam
Vinblastine
    delirium due to, 62

depression due to, 76
Vincristine
    constipation due to, 56
    delirium due to, 62
    depression due to, 76
VIPoma, diarrhea due to, 97
Viral infection, in AIDS patients, diarrhea due to, 97
Viscous lidocaine, for mucositis, 158t
Vistaril. *See* Hydroxyzine
Visual analog scale, in depression diagnosis, 77
Vitamin E, for mucositis, 158t
    oral, 147
Vomiting, nausea and, in palliative care patients, 163-181. *See also* Nausea and vomiting, in palliative care patients

Wald, F., 4
Weakness, constipation due to, 50
Weight loss, significant, megestrol acetate in patients with, 19
Welbutin. *See* Bupropion
White light, for depression, 74t
World Health Organization (WHO), palliative care definition by, 3
Worthlessness, feelings of, depression and, 76

Xanax. *See* Alprazolam
Xerostomia (dry mouth)
    drugs and, 188
    in palliative care patients
        causes of, 149
        defined, 149
        drugs and, 151-153
    in palliative care patients, 146,151-153
Xylocaine. *See* Lidocaine

Zollinger-Ellison disease, diarrhea due to, 97
Zoloft. *See* Sertraline